Contents

It is Different

Christmas Eve 2006

It is different. It looks different. It feels different. I must be imagining it. I don't want to think about it – I am so frightened and scared stiff really. What if it is? It just seems a bit swollen, a bit granular, on just one side. No one will believe me. No one will take me seriously. What do I tell my husband Andy? I can't tell him yet. I need to be sure first. We don't have secrets, but this is one and I feel so scared and guilty for not telling him.

It is 11.30am on Christmas Eve and Dad is travelling down from Cheshire on his own again for our second Christmas without Mum. I couldn't tell him if my worst fears came true – I think it would destroy him, he would be devastated. How would he cope again? Here he is now – we must enjoy our quiet Christmas together.

'Merry Christmas Dad'

Thursday 27th December

We have had a very quiet and relaxing Christmas Day and Boxing Day. We have eaten far too much, watched too much TV, opened loads of wonderful presents and enjoyed the quiet time together as a threesome with Chloe, our black Labrador dog. Bliss for a while; then back it comes to the forefront of my mind. I do miss Mum – it isn't the same since she died. She was so wonderful, calm and bright, and always there for me. Always worried about how hard I worked. What would she think if it came true... if it is the same? She was always so positive and a fighter. She is my inspiration and I miss her so much.

I have just had a bath before bedtime, which is my idea of sheer luxury and total relaxation. Absolute heaven really and where I hope to escape that feeling. It is still different. I need to stop checking. I need to think of something else. I am imagining it? It can't be the worst – I am too well. I do get very tired but apart from my thyroid problem, and aches and pains with my back and neck, I am doing OK for a 52 year old. I just can't tell Andy – he will think I am silly!

New Year's Day 2007

Fabulous New Year's Eve – met at a Chinese restaurant with our closest friends Andy and Karon, Bob and Dot, and Pauline and Roger. It was a great atmosphere and fabulous food. We all ate too much and because Andy was driving home there was lots of wine for me.

The New Year's Gala Evening Concert at Symphony Hall in Birmingham was fabulous; super classics, with party poppers, balloons and paper bags to burst in tune to the 1812 overture. Rule Britannia, Jerusalem and Land of Hope and Glory were fantastic, great fun, extremely well performed and just the ticket for bringing in a New Year.

Everyone wishes each other a Happy New Year and we kiss and hug each other at midnight. I hate that moment really, the painting, a façade, as I have always been scared of what an unknown New Year could bring after the Millennium brought Alan losing his battle and in 2005 Mum losing her battle too.

I hope my silly thoughts, neurotic feelings and extra sensitivity are nothing to be concerned about – probably just my total imagination.

Wednesday 3rd January

I returned to work yesterday and worked in the office and at home to get myself sorted out for the very busy half term ahead. I work for the Local Authority as a School Adviser and tomorrow schools return from their break, and with it the return of a rapid increase in e-mail messages, phone calls and appointments, as it is our core business time with the schools.

My ongoing back and neck joint problems really cause me so many aches and pains, which I have learnt to manage by regularly attending the rehab gym at the chiropractor clinic, including having regular manipulation (tweaking as I call it!). Recently I have had lots of aches and pains since Chloe got excited with two other dogs and set off my joints when I firmly got hold of her! Off to the chiropractor now and then I will feel much better after a fragile 36 hours. The appointment is at 4pm – I need to allow 50 minutes to get there from work and then it is 25 minutes to drive home for some pampering. Oh bath here I come.

Saturday 6th January

Just had a wonderful lazy bath and washed my hair to get dressed up for Wendy and Clive to arrive for dinner. I have spent the afternoon preparing the meal.

It still looks different, still feels different, and is about as granular as before. I still think I am imagining it and being over-sensitive and neurotic too. I can't tell Andy, as I am so scared and frightened – what if it really is my worst nightmare coming true? How on earth would I face it and find the strength to do so?

Tuesday 9th January

Andy has left to go to Luton airport to fly to Turin until Thursday evening. It is his first trip to Turin for the motor company he has been working for since mid October. At least it is only two nights and Europe rather than eight nights in India, which he did in December. Chloe and I miss him but we manage everything and do lots of dog walking either side of work – even in the dark along the unlit country lanes carrying a torch.

I am still worried, it still seems the same, hasn't miraculously disappeared as hoped: still different and granular. It must be something – I just don't know what to do. If only Andy was here!

Thursday 18th January

It has been a really busy day at work today and a busy week too. I planned and led a very important meeting with secondary schools on Monday about teaching and learning developments in ICT (Information and Communication Technology – computers basically) and implementation of another government target. Attendance was excellent with nearly forty teachers and Headteachers. It went really well – the exuberance though, didn't take away how stressed and tired I felt when I got home.

This morning I had to do a fifteen-minute presentation on the same topic to seventy primary Headteachers at their monthly briefing. Even though my preparation was thorough my nerves kicked in, but as I stood up my confidence came back when I could see the audience did not see my underlying fears. It seemed to go well.

Later I relaxed in the bath before bed to de-stress, unwind and chill out. I am still really worried… I am sure it is a bit bigger, and slightly more granular. I know I should go to the doctors. I am so frightened it is the same problem that Mum had which ultimately claimed her life in August 2005.

Saturday 20th January

I am getting neurotic, over-sensitive and pre-occupied. I'm beginning to wonder if I really do have a problem because it hasn't miraculously gone away as I wished. I'll check again when I have bath tonight, before I go with Andy to a classical music concert and a meal out afterwards. I won't tell him tonight as it will only spoil the evening and we get very little precious time together anyway.

Tuesday 23rd January

I have just had my bath before bed, which I so enjoy at the end of another extremely busy day. The job just gets bigger, broader and more intense and everyday is just frantic, hectic and demands 'mental gymnastics' in order to survive.

I have checked myself — it is still the same, still granular and still feels different. But I can't explain why, I feel such a fraud. I really should go to the doctors for peace of mind. I must build up my courage and confront this. I really must tell Andy — I know he will order me to the doctors.

I have just told Andy my worst fears. Tears streamed down my face because I am so very frightened. He is as logical, straight forward and as pragmatic as ever and makes me realise that if I think I have a problem then I must go to the doctors to get it checked for peace of mind. I do know this but I just don't want to face it.

Testing times

Wednesday 24th January

I have telephoned the doctor's surgery this morning to make an appointment for 5.20pm. I feel better now I have done it. I expect he will send me home and tell me not to worry as he can't find anything. I text Andy to let him know I have made the appointment and to check he will be home to walk Chloe whilst I am at the doctors. He is pleased I have made the move.

The doctor checks me over and agrees it does feel different, not a lump, a bit granular and perhaps slightly fuller. He is not supposed to agree with me! I am a bit worried now. He tries to reassure me by saying he wouldn't be worried if I was his wife, but he will refer me to a consultant to be checked anyway, due to my family history.

I leave home at 7pm to go to a leaving meal for a

colleague at an Indian restaurant. It is a great evening but my mind is a little muddled really. Thanks for little mercies that colleagues have no idea of my thoughts.

Thursday 25th January

As we have private medical insurance with Andy's job we decide to use the benefit. I telephoned the doctor today to acquire the name of a Consultant for Breast Surgery at the Private Hospital, which fortunately is about 20 minutes from home. I rang the hospital at 2.30pm and was given an appointment at 6.30pm tomorrow (Friday evening) – great end to a busy week – but thankfully really soon. I text Andy with the time and he instantly says he will attend with me – just what I hoped he would do and knew in my heart that he would want to anyway.

Friday 26th January

I gave a presentation about the ICT development twice today – at 9am to Headteachers of special schools and again at 2.30pm to 50 Local Authority Advisory Service colleagues to keep them in the picture of the developments with schools. Both events went really well and everyone says how helpful, clear and to the point the presentation was overall. They now feel up-to-date and understand what the next steps will be and how they can support the work of the Local Authority when in schools.

In the back of my mind I'm hoping the rest of my day will go as well.

We arrive at 6.30pm for the consultant appointment at the hospital and see the Consultant at 6.40pm. He asks lots of questions – why I am there, about my family medical history and my own medical history. He reads the doctor's letter of referral. He then examines me and I expect him to tell me to go home.

No he doesn't: 'You are right it does feel different.' He isn't supposed to say that. I think to myself 'Oh, shit!' 'We need to do a mammogram and ultra sound scan – now – down the corridor.'

I get dressed and ask if Andy can go with us. The nurse leading me walks so fast down the corridor that the pace of my concern speeds up with her. The radiographer asks me to change into a gown and then takes four images of each breast; two from the side and two from the top looking downwards. It is always painful for those few seconds when they squeeze the flesh between the plates to take the images. She asks me to wait for a few minutes whilst she checks the images are as she wants them. While I am sitting there in my gown I begin to feel even more scared and worried. This shouldn't be happening to me.

I am then taken into another hospital room for an ultra sound scan of both breasts and surrounding areas. The gel they use is really cold. Time seems to hang in the air and 40 minutes later we are back in the consulting room.

Based upon the results of the mammogram I would be sent home with no further treatment, as it looks clear! However, the radiographer is very concerned about the ultra sound scan results. I am not really surprised, as he seemed to spend ages scanning my right breast area, taking lots of images.

'It could be cancer.' I hear myself reply 'Right – but if it isn't what could it be?'

'It could be abnormal cells, or unstable and pre-cancerous cells or cancer – any way we would be better removing it to check fully.'

I am beginning to get shocked and frightened. My worst nightmare is staring me in the face.

'The next step is to complete a needle biopsy and if you get on the bed we'll do that now!'

It is so painful and like large chopsticks being inserted into the flesh and then twisted around. It leaves a huge bruise for a week!

'Come back at 12.30pm on Monday and we'll have the results; meanwhile go home, take two pain killing tablets and have a glass of wine.'

Andy replies from the other side of the curtain. 'The bottle is already in the fridge!' That briefly puts a smile on my face.

We are stunned, shocked and in disbelief sitting in the car, one hour and ten minutes after arriving. What a weekend to get through!

Saturday 27th January

The weekend is very tense and worrying yet relaxing too as we stay at Andy and Karon's (with Chloe) for a wine tasting evening with friends. I have to tell them about the pressure and worry we are both under so they understand why I may not be as bright as usual. It was a great tonic and just the entertainment and super companionship for a stressful weekend. Karon is like a sister to me and so lovely. We arrived home at 2pm on Sunday when the worry took over again and thoughts of what to do next came to the fore.

I rang Jack my line manager on Saturday, so he would know what pressure I am under. He agrees to visit a secondary school on Monday afternoon on my behalf whilst I am at the hospital for the biopsy results.

Monday 29th January

I arrive at work at 8.10am ready to set up for a training session for ICT teachers. Rachel and Carl, who I line manage, are delivering most of the day anyway. I am delivering a presentation, which is the introduction from 9.00 - 9.30am. This goes well and the course is well on the way. I tell Rachel and Carl that I have been called to an important meeting and will need to leave at 11 o'clock rather than at lunchtime. I just can't tell them why – they don't suspect anything.

Andy and I arrive at home from work and set off together to go to the hospital. I think the most difficult and nervous meeting of my life. Andy feels the same but we hold hands as we walk in ten minutes early. They are ready for us and in we go.

'Based upon the biopsy results it is pre-cancerous, unstable and we believe not cancer.'

The relief is enormous!

'It is in the lobular tissue rather than the milk ducts, which explains why the mammogram didn't pick it up.'

That's worrying as my letter for a three-year screening appointment arrived at lunchtime and is for 23rd February. The Consultant makes it clear that he will remove the unstable tissue in a wide local excision operation on Wednesday. A full biopsy will determine the extent and exact problem – he is very optimistic it is contained and no further treatment will be needed. We just need that result for an absolute all clear.

I ring Dad and explain. I chose not to tell him when I rang on Saturday, as I didn't want to worry him unduly.

He is shocked, supportive and glad it is pre-cancerous rather than cancer. This is all he needs after losing Mum from breast cancer in 2005 and Alan (my twin brother) from bowel cancer in May 2000, after a five year battle against the disease.

Tuesday 30th January

I go into work today to sort myself out as I hope to be back next week, and put all of this behind us. There is a lot to sort out and key people to see. I tell my immediate colleagues about my scare and surgery. Jack knows and is totally supportive. I inform members of my advisory team and ICT technicians – at least the few who are in the building, as many are out visiting schools.

This is too close a call. I never want to be here again. It does look optimistic. It does look like I have caught it early. A legacy from Mum and a positive outcome of her death from breast cancer is that I check and examine myself so carefully – could say neurotically! I took her advice. Bless her.

I leave work expecting to return in a week at the latest, although we are still cautious about being over joyful until a full biopsy is completed after the operation. We are due to get the results next Wednesday when the stitches will also be removed.

Everyone wishes me well and is so supportive. I meet

Rebecca (Head of Service) in the corridor. She is choked when I explain about my weekend of worry. She has known me since I have lost Alan and Mum and therefore is very concerned and scared for me.

Mount Everest

Wednesday 31st January

I starve myself from 7.30am ready to be in hospital at 12.30pm. Andy goes to work and leaves early to return home for 11.00am to drive me to the hospital. He is wonderful. His new work colleagues are being supportive too and allowing him to take any time he needs to be with me.

We arrive on time and I am admitted. We go through the medical questions numerous times, as all of the staff are very thorough. We are very impressed with their quality of care and speed of treatment. When I come around from the operation, I am so sore and feel weird. Andy has gone home to take Chloe for a walk and will come and collect me later. He is calm and strong. I do love him.

We arrive home at 8.30pm. I am very tired, sore and

sleepy. Andy helps me to get undressed and I have a reasonable night's sleep because of the painkilling tablets.

Saturday 3rd February

I am making good progress overall. My wound is a bit sore but with the painkillers it is bearable. I slept most of yesterday, which I think was the effect of the anaesthetic. Andy is great, doing some of the jobs and looking after me when I need it.

We are still optimistic, but just feel we can't open the champagne until we get the absolute all clear next Wednesday. It should be OK; I hope it is OK; this has been close enough as it is! Karon texts me messages of support each day. She is fabulous and so strong for me. She has had a few scares herself so understands what I am going through.

Monday 5th February

I was hoping to be back at work today but I feel too tired and a bit sore. I've decided to go back on Thursday and Friday, after I have seen the Consultant again. It is the school half term holiday then for a week, so life can get back to normal afterwards. I'll visit the doctor tomorrow as my first ever seven days off work will be up and I need a sick note to cover my absence so that my pay isn't affected. This is a new experience for me, because I have never had more than four consecutive days off before. I will certainly be glad when we are given the all clear. Wednesday can't come soon enough, but I am a bit scared because knowing my luck it will not be clear and my worst nightmare really will come true.

Wednesday 7th February

My stitches are removed today and I hope it won't be painful. Andy and I are concerned we may not get the all clear, from the biopsy on the cells removed last week. The Consultant was very optimistic, but obviously covering himself really. All the fabulous e-mail messages from work, including Jack and Emma (my secretary), say 'they wish me luck and have their fingers crossed for me'.

Andy gets home late morning so he can go to the hospital with me. He is so supportive. He is optimistic, strong, a bit apprehensive but hoping to open the champagne tonight. I am hoping too – I am scared now.

We arrive, and when called in, the Consultant Nurse for Breast Care is present, with the Consultant. He starts to explain that 'the biopsy shows there are cancer cells on the outer face of the flesh they have removed and they need to do further surgery which will include removing the lymph nodes in the arm pit'. As he explains and we start to ask questions it suddenly dawns on me, that it is invasive breast cancer and not pre-cancerous cells as we thought. I am stunned, start to feel upset and cry a bit.

Andy looks near to tears and bowled over too. He is strong though and helps me by asking lots of questions about the prognosis and the next steps. Many can't be answered yet until we have a clear picture of the cancer after the next stage.

I will be given a choice of a second wide local excision and lymph node removal or full reconstruction mastectomy – only a 45 minute operation compared with five hours of major surgery! The Nurse will explain all of this to us on Friday, once we have had time to absorb today's news. I will also have chemotherapy and radiotherapy offered to me. This is now a nightmare!

I really didn't think I would be facing all of this; it is so scary, huge, nightmarish, frightening, and life changing! Suddenly I feel I have been whipped up by a tornado onto another road or track for my life's destiny. No more work for months – how do you cope with that! I am the sort of person who has to keep active. What will happen to all my hard work over the years?

We arrive at home. We hug and cry in a state of shock. We feel absolutely stunned, as if we have been crushed by a huge steamroller. In some ways the turmoil sensation is like a sudden bereavement. We take Chloe for a long walk to try and talk and come to terms with the news. I ring Dad, which is one of the hardest calls I have ever made in my life. He takes it well but says he feels guilty because of Alan too. I reassure him that he shouldn't; no one knows why both twins have cancer and their Mum too. I hope I survive as Alan and Mum didn't - I can't afford to think like that at all. I have got to be positive; that is extremely hard at the moment. I feel someone has said, 'Well you have coped fine with the past; now let us see how you deal with Mount Everest right in front of you.' *'Bugger!'* My only word for the disease before this happened and now a triple *'bugger'*.

Thursday 8th February

The weather has turned foul overnight and it has dumped four inches of snow outside. I am glad I am signed off from work and haven't got to struggle in. Andy emails his work and lets them know he needs to spend time with me to come to terms with the news and talk about the next steps. They are fine about it all.

We spend the day pottering about doing things, hugging a lot, talking when we want to and just being together. I would hate to have to cope with this without Andy – in fact I know I couldn't. I rang Jack too, late yesterday afternoon, and he will have told my main Adviser colleagues, Rebecca and my team. I agree the best form of communication is by email rather than phone, if people wish to get in touch.

I just couldn't text the news to Karon. Instead I left her a text asking her to phone me when she could, so I could fill her in. When she did, she was stunned and her immediate reaction was 'shit!' I know what she means and Andy has used that word a lot in the last twenty-four hours – 'a really shitty day' was his summary. I couldn't agree more.

Friday 9th February

Andy stays at home from work again, as we are due at the hospital to talk to the Consultant Nurse about the surgery options. They will want my decision by ten o'clock on Monday morning in order to schedule the surgery. Things are moving incredibly fast.

We arrive with numerous questions including some about the chemotherapy. The Nurse explains she wants to focus upon the surgery today so that I am fully informed in order to make my decision over the weekend. She will talk to us about chemotherapy on Monday, rather than bombarding us with details. We are having the information in chunks in order to absorb it and take it all in. It is mind blowing and so frightening really. Is this really happening to me? Why is it happening to me at all?

The surgery details are very scary; the major surgery makes my stomach turn at the thought of it. The photos of the final outcome from a full reconstruction mastectomy do look good, although the thought of the pain, stitches, drains and five weeks recovery is so frightening. They use fat and muscle from your stomach area to rebuild the breast. Yuk. If the success rate for both operations is the same, my initial thoughts are the 45 minute operation is well worth a try. Removal of the lymph nodes sounds daunting enough, and I remember about the risk of lymphoedema and long term care required from my Mum's experience.

We go home after another hour and a half meeting. We have so much to absorb and think about. I feel less stressed and calmer; and know I have to face this reality now. I needed to know all the facts and the next steps to start the journey up the mountain. It seems such a massive mountain in front of me at the moment.

Saturday 10th February

It seems a long time since Wednesday. I have telephoned a few friends who are all very stunned and so supportive. I can just about talk about it without getting too upset. They are wonderful. We need them to help us to get through this.

Andy and I are both becoming calmer, talking more about our future, what we should do, and the next steps. It is so incredibly hard and very frightening to comprehend that I may not survive this cancer as we don't yet have a prognosis. We are stunned, upset at times, happy together hugging and kissing, and in love even more. This certainly takes some getting your head around. Why? What have I done to deserve it? Why three of us out of four in my family? What would my Mum and Alan think? Dad still feels guilty but I think he is coping reasonably well.

We keep talking about the surgery choices and I think I have made up my mind really. I decide not to ask any friends or family for their opinions and don't tell them which way I will go. Andy listens to me whenever I need to talk it through and has agreed he will support me what ever I decide to do. It is my choice; I am the one who has to go through the surgery; I am the one facing this nightmare and whose life is in the balance.

Monday 12th February

We arrive for our appointment and I inform the Nurse of my decision to try the wide local excision and lymph node operation. I do fully understand that if it is not successful at removing the cancer, then the mastectomy operation would be the next step. They then book me into hospital for Wednesday, which is Valentine's Day – how romantic!

I do feel relieved that I have a way forward in this nightmare. At last it is a first positive step in the battle and the journey up the Mountain. I have now become much calmer; less short tempered; less stunned, and ready to face and tackle the reality. It isn't easy though but Andy is with me totally.

We talk to the Nurse for another hour and a half. Most

things are very clear and she is so supportive and knowledgeable. She spends ages explaining the chemotherapy and radiotherapy. I will be given one dose of the first drug every three weeks times four for stage 1, which makes twelve weeks in total. This will then be followed by stage 2! I will then be given three drugs on week one and two and then no drugs for week three and four (i.e. a four-week cycle). This will be repeated four times, which is a total of sixteen weeks in stage 2. This means the chemotherapy is administered for nearly seven months! This seems a lifetime. Seven months of treatment takes some grasping and coming to terms with too. The future looks so bleak and the treatment sounds horrendous. It will be nearly a whole year of my life having treatment for cancer. What a nightmare.

It really upsets me to realise I will lose my hair – not partially or thinning, but completely within two to three weeks of the start of treatment. This takes some dealing with in the time-scale, as I knew it would be months of chemotherapy from what Mum went through, but I thought the hair loss came later – in July or August. I am not looking forward to being bald at all. The Nurse gives us valuable advice about wigs, scarves and hats. We are given a catalogue and details of a recommended wig shop to go to in the next few weeks if I decide to wear one. She also gives us a scarf for me to try at home and practical suggestions on how to wear it. I just can't comprehend the thought of how I will look bald, and how on earth I will face the world and everyone I meet at work.

She told us that the Oncologist does encourage patients to get on with their lives, but to listen to their bodies during the chemotherapy months. He does allow certain patients to return to work on a part-time basis as well. This cheers me up as I think I would like to do that to ensure I keep on top of things and also to give me a sense of purpose for getting out of bed. Like I've said, I'm the sort of person that needs to be active. It would also provide some normality in this long period of treatment.

Chemotherapy would start two to six weeks after surgery. So if the operation on Wednesday is successful – I certainly hope it is – then I could be having treatment and my hair would be gone before Easter. I'm not sure I can take the rapidity of all of this in. Andy feels everything is a whirlwind too. We are mentally, emotionally, physically drained and exhausted when we get home. Everyday is mind blowing! It is so tough to absorb but we will get through this – I am determined.

Friends and family are telephoning and being really wonderful. I can comfortably talk about it without getting upset now, which helps us all. Work colleagues have also been emailing me supportive messages. It makes me cry when I read them as they too are in shock and can't believe this is happening to me. The main advantage of email is that when I am in tears replying, they can't see that side of me. I am very positive and upbeat in the replies, because that is how I want to convey this experience and I guess most of the time that is how I am beginning to feel anyway.

Tuesday 13th February

I went into work today to see Jack and Emma. I discussed who could cover which aspects of my job in my absence, and sorted out my emails and desk. It was hard walking in but as it is half term very few colleagues were in the building, so it was easier than it could have been.

Jack is supportive and really doesn't want me to worry. I know I have to put myself first. I was able to let him know what the Consultant Nurse told us yesterday; 'that the Oncologist encourages you to work and lead a normal life during chemotherapy', so I may be back part time fairly soon. That should help the Service and give me something to aim for too. It was extremely hard walking out and I was upset as I hugged them goodbye, as I am not sure exactly when I will be returning to work in the future.

Romantic Valentine's Day

Wednesday 14th February

Andy usually doesn't remember Valentine's Day but he delights me with a new moth orchid plant to add to my collection in the kitchen. It is lovely and so unlike him. I have bought him an Elephant soft toy with 'love you lots' on his tummy.

I am booked into hospital at 12 noon and go to theatre at one o'clock. I will be in hospital for two or three nights and will have a drain attached to the lymph node area for the fluids to drain away. I'm not looking forward to that at all.

As Andy and I walk hand-in-hand up the hospital steps in silence, I can see the anxiety on his face. When he glanced back at me he just smiled and squeezed my hand tighter as if to say 'we'll get over that mountain.' Andy helps me get prepared and reassures me by giving me a kiss and a hug. I put on a brave smile but to be honest I just feel numb with the anxiety of the operation.

When I come around I am so tired but don't feel in too much pain as I am on pain killing tablets. Andy visits me after going home and walking Chloe whilst I am in the operating theatre. The nurse rang him to confirm I had come through the operation and anaesthetic OK. Apparently Chloe is confused – she isn't the only one!

Thursday 15th February

I have had a reasonable night but my lymph node wound really hurts this morning as the local anaesthetic they applied has now worn off. I have to take regular tablets to ease the pain. Numerous people come in and out of the room during the morning – nurses, duty doctors, catering staff, cleaners, physiotherapist, pharmacist, the Consultant Nurse, and the Consultant who performed the operation. Some of them come in several times. It is like being in Piccadilly Circus.

I am getting used to carrying my drain around with me – the six-foot tube with body fluid in isn't a pretty sight really. I was advised to bring in a draw string sponge bag to cover the bottle so that does help the look immensely! The nurses are fabulous. I have to loose any inhibitions when they have to take you to the bathroom for the first 24 hours to check that you are OK (with the drain carried in the sponge bag). It is hard and painful to wash myself too so they have to help me with my left underarm, legs and feet. Getting the elastic stockings on and off is a challenge for them and a huge embarrassment for me.

Andy and Karon squeeze in a visit to see me, in between their trip to see the Northern lights and a weekend in London. They are such great friends and Karon spoils me with lots of little presents. The little white bear she gives me ends up on my bed being cuddled as a comforter. Andy comes out of work to have his lunch with me. It is so great to see him and talk to him. I miss him and Chloe.

Friday 16th February

I am making good progress overall and everyone is pleased with me. The physiotherapist visits again to check I am doing the arm exercises to stretch the lymph node area. It is painful but essential to prevent swelling and lymphoedema and to get the flexibility back too. They send me for an x-ray and an ultra sound scan at 1.00pm. They are checking the liver, chest wall cavity, bone density and breast area for any spread of the cancer. I am suddenly extremely scared – what if the results this afternoon are positive – that will be really bad news.

I eventually get my lunch at 1.45pm after starving from 8.00am for the scan. This was much later than I thought it would be and even though I knew I would get the results this afternoon it still seemed a long time. Our friend Liz visited me for about half an hour as she has had an appointment at the hospital and knew I would still be recovering from the operation. It was a nice relief to see someone I could talk to and not a member of the medical profession and certainly helped to take my mind off the impending results.

The results are all clear – what a relief and this adds to a positive picture. I hope the operation is also successful in removing the cancer and I don't have to face the mastectomy surgery at all.

It is decided at four o'clock that I can go home later as I am only resting and waiting for the fluid in the drain to be clear, which apparently could take until Monday or even next Wednesday. I text Andy and he collects me at 7.30pm after the Nurse has checked my dressing and sorted me out with my drain and tube still attached.

Saturday 17th February

It is good to be home and Andy has the weekend to look after me. He has to help me wash in the bath as I can only sit in it, because the dressings have to be kept dry. He helps me change my elastic stockings, and to get them back on too, as they have to be worn for 24 hours a day. I have to wear them for at least a week – Oh what joy! We struggled to get them on this morning and just as we thought we had succeeded, I realised they were on inside out! We had to start all over again but we certainly laughed about it.

Jack rings from work to see how I am, which is really kind of him. Bob and Dot ring and come over for a while. It is lovely to see them but I am very tired when they leave and I go straight to bed. Chloe is happier now I am home. She wagged her tail in excitement and brought me one of her favourite toys in her mouth when I came through the door. She knew that things weren't right and really fretted for me.

Monday 19th February

I have telephoned the Nurse each day as arranged to let her know how the fluid in the drain is progressing. She is pleased and thinks we should see her at nine o'clock to have it removed. When we arrive I thought at least one of the men sitting in reception was going to pass out seeing this tube (and sponge bag) with body fluids in attached to me and placed next to my chair! The drain is removed and it is such a relief, I feel so free now. I am progressing well. Andy takes more time off work so he can go to the hospital with me. We have four days there this week!

Tuesday 20th February

Andy is at work today – a full day for a change. Dad and my mother-in-law Joyce came down from Nantwich to see me. They arrived at 11.30am and left at 6.00pm after Andy was home from work. It was good to catch up. They are both angry and cross about what has happened to me, but supportive and cheerful. I had a rest on the bed for an hour and half to cope with the day, which did help. They brought the pudding and some of the food for tea to make it easier for me. Dad seems to be coping quite well, although he does still feel guilty, which he shouldn't at all – it isn't his fault. He seems to think it is genetic. I don't know whether it is or not. Will we ever know?

Wednesday 21st February

Andy arrives home from work at eleven o'clock again to take me for the biopsy results with the Consultant at 12.30pm. It is another Wednesday – I am either going in for surgery or having results on a Wednesday – it is such a key day. I am beginning to dread Wednesdays.

When we are sitting in reception the Consultant Nurse comes along to collect us and is really excited. She can't contain herself, and tells us as we step through the door that it is good news. The Consultant explains that the operation has been successful, they have removed all of the cancer (even though it was a 5.2 centimetre area in total) and the cancer is only in one lymph node out of the nine removed. This is very good news indeed apparently. Less than four affected lymph nodes are statistically curable and case studies prove this out. Thank goodness!

The blood vessels that cross the cancer cells haven't been invaded either – more positives. I am also suitable for a well known oestrogen receptor antagonist drug i.e. blocker, for oestrogen based cancers like mine. This is very positive news and I don't mind at all having to take one tablet a day for the next five years. We are delighted and I am especially pleased that I don't need to face the five hours of surgery for the mastectomy reconstruction. I am overwhelmingly relieved. This is the best news we have had in four weeks – things are looking good. I might outlive Chloe now (who is only four years old) and also enjoy my early retirement plans with Andy. It is strange how you think of these things when you are scared and in a serious life-threatening situation. We telephoned Dad and Joyce and family and friends and naturally they are all really pleased for us.

Being cruel to be kind

Thursday 22nd February

As I don't need any more surgery for the cancer, it is an appointment with the Oncologist this morning to discuss the chemotherapy treatment. He is very thorough with his questions and in examining me. He is impressed with my health and muscle tone around my neck, shoulders and stomach. This is accounted for by my workouts at the gym for my neck, back and shoulder problems and in order to build strength in those areas. So far these problems have been fine throughout the last four weeks – time will tell.

Apparently the anaesthetist has advised that I would be better having a small metal device and line inserted to use for all blood samples and injections of the chemotherapy. This is because my veins in the hand are so poor and very difficult to find. I would only struggle extensively every visit. It is decided to operate next Wednesday, stay in overnight and then have the first chemotherapy early Thursday morning.

When we get in the car we are stunned again at the whirlwind speed of the treatment. They do not hang about and we cannot fault the team of specialists, and the quality of service we are receiving.

Thursday 23rd February

We are at the hospital for the fourth day this week – Andy has been with me every-time and taken time out of work for it. They have been superb about it all and we are so grateful. The car knows its' own way to the hospital now!

I have the stitches removed by the Consultant Nurse and she is really pleased with the healing of the scars and my arm movements when getting undressed and dressed again. I am doing my exercises every day as instructed, but they do hurt and stretching is sore. No wonder when the incision across the actual armpit is about two and half inches (twelve centimetres) long, and my scar on my right breast is also two inches long (ten centimetres).

Saturday 24th February

The doorbell rang at about three o'clock. It was Mo, one of my neighbours who stood there and said 'Is it true?' She had heard from one of the neighbours that Andy had seen when out walking Chloe. Mo stopped for a coffee and was very supportive and concerned. She totally understands as she had breast cancer herself eight years ago and underwent the same treatment. I enjoyed her visit and think she will be a great mentor and inspiration to me throughout the next few months.

Our friends Barry and Lillian came over for a couple of hours and the men fetched a Chinese takeaway meal. The meal was fun, with good food, plenty of wine and a big laugh, which certainly helped. It was a lovely evening and so easy to do with very little preparation.

Tuesday 27th February

I visited the doctor today to renew my sick note for work. We decide 27th March is probably best for me to return to work. So I have three to four weeks to get over all of the surgery and also get through to the second three-week cycle of chemotherapy. I can see how I am before considering part time work. At least it is giving me a target and a time-scale to aim for which is motivating. The four walls at home are beginning to get tedious now. I am also very fed-up with daytime television programmes!

Wednesday 28th February

I feel a bit low this week as it is a shame that I have to have a third anaesthetic in a four-week period, to have the implant device inserted, which is more stitches and more recovery. I suppose it is being cruel to be kind really! The device is the size of a bottle top with a membrane cover. It is inserted under the skin during the surgery and has a fine tube attached which they thread through the chest to a heart vein so that the drugs will go into the blood stream and they also have easy access for taking blood samples. They have to implant it to the left of my left breast just below the armpit in the fatty tissue, as they can't use the right side because of the cancerous area.

I am admitted at 12 noon after starving myself again from eight o'clock. Surgery is at two o'clock and it is only a 20 minute operation. The anaesthetist has trouble finding a vein in the back of my hand (what a surprise!) and inserts it in the inside of the elbow instead. I suppose this proves why I need the device for future use. Chemotherapy involves twelve doses of drugs and twelve blood tests over seven months – such a long process and time. This means I will be on treatment until September and then it is three and a half weeks of daily visits for radiotherapy. This seems never ending, but hopefully it is the insurance policy for my future life and our happy retirement together.

Thursday 1st March

I had a terrible night's sleep, as there is an extractor fan system outside the bedroom window that constantly switches on and off. The clock ticks so loudly too, adding to my aggravation. I am so nervous and worried about the chemotherapy. My sister-in-law Gill (Alan's widow) sent me text messages of support which helped keep me calm.

The Oncologist and specialist oncology nurse arrive in my room at 7.10am (he starts work at seven o'clock and likes his patients to arrive for treatment and consultation at 7.30am!). He examines me thoroughly and is pleased with everything. My blood samples are taken to check that the blood count and platelet levels are high enough for the treatment. My blood samples are taken at 7.20am using the newly implanted device and the oncology nurse arrived at 8.10am with the chemotherapy drugs. These are in a sealed and labelled case. She also has a saline drip on a stand. She attaches a plastic syringe link to the inserted device in my left side and chats to me as I eat breakfast whilst she pumps in at least four huge syringes of bright pink fluid. It is painless but a bit daunting and takes about 25 minutes. I am able to text Andy at nine o'clock to ask him to collect me to take me home.

Friday 2nd March

I slept like a baby in my own bed last night. I am so tired and relieved I am now on the long, steady ascent up the mountain after having made some huge strides in the last four weeks. I am sore but things are manageable – I only have four wounds and two dressings on now! (One on the right breast; one in the right armpit; one to the left of my left breast including a half-inch incision in my chest which is to secure the line internally to my heart vein.)

Andy enjoys the weekend looking after me and I sleep most of the time due I think to the relief at this stage – or is it the chemotherapy? I only have to take nine tablets at breakfast time, six at lunchtime, five at teatime, and four at bedtime – not many at all! So far they do seem to stop me feeling sick.

Monday 5th March

I am feeling a lot less tired today. The only problem is constipation (from the painkillers and steroids) and I have to resort to sachets to sort my system out. Also I am starting to get heartburn, which is really painful. I'll have to talk to them about this next time. It says on the label you can't take any other indigestion remedies whilst on these tablets. We'll see how I go. I am drinking my two litres of water a day as advised to flush the drugs through the system. I am constantly weeing too!

Andy has taken a day's leave today and is working on the bathroom renovation project. It is good relaxation after the upheaval of the last few weeks. We both feel calmer, more relaxed, much closer than ever and valuing each other tremendously.

I have been doing a lot of thinking since the Nurse

explained about the wigs, scarves and hats that I could wear. I know in my heart that I do not want to look like a cancer patient if I can avoid it. I strongly believe that when you see a lady wearing a scarf or hat with no hair showing it is obvious that she is undergoing chemotherapy treatment. I hate the very thought of going out in public without any hair and everyone staring at me and knowing that I am battling with cancer. Even the notion of being bald at home in private makes my stomach turn. I have made up my mind to be strong and determined about this and to try and buy a wig that is very natural looking so that I can wear it all the time. Neither am I keen on wearing scarves or hats in public. If I can achieve this natural look then I will be able to function much better at work too. As an Adviser I visit lots of schools and attend many meetings. Most importantly I plan and deliver training for teachers at the Office base, which has training facilities. When I stand up in front of an audience I would feel more normal and most people wouldn't know I was on treatment. Even if they knew I could at least look healthy and blend in with everyone in the room. I suppose some people would think this was silly and not important but it is my way of dealing with this trauma and radical treatment period. They aren't the ones losing their hair in a few days time!

Tuesday 6th March

I decided to keep my dental check up appointment today at nine o'clock. I did feel terrible driving there – all hot and weak and in some pain too. At least I am now checked for six months. I am not allowed to see the hygienist as they don't want any bleeding of the gums as apparently this can allow infection in which can be dangerous whilst on chemotherapy. I won't miss those appointments at all.

I then moved my car to another car park and wandered around a department store looking for some casual clothes. It was an effort and I thought I was going to pass out at the checkout queue. I am really suffering with hot flushes, which makes me feel worse. The Oncology Nurse has suggested taking sage oil tablets to try and help with these. I was really glad to collapse and rest when I got home. I think all the pills in a morning make me feel weird and then they wear off during the day. I only started chemotherapy a few days ago, which must be having an effect on my body – probably in ways I don't understand yet.

Wednesday 7th March

Andy has taken a day's leave so that we can go to a shop recommended by the Consultant Nurse to choose this important wig so that I am ready for when my hair falls out in about ten days time. Not the best way to spend a day's leave but we have a leisurely 45 minute drive across country from the motorway and arrive early. The lady assistant is so professional and discrete. You are in a private room, so it isn't as bad as we thought it could be.

I tried five wigs on and quickly chose one that is light brown, with highlights of a paler shade, so it looks quite blonde. It is also longer in the neck than my current hairstyle. My hair is horrible at the moment anyway, as it is flat, lank, shorter than usual, and should have had a perm applied two weeks ago. That would have been a waste of money. I suppose that is one way of looking at it.

I feel pleased with the wig and we buy a brush, and special shampoo and conditioner. I also chose three scarves, which I can wear around the house or in the garden when the weather is hot. Two of them are floral with plain elastic bands and ties that drape down your back. They are quite pretty and in my favourite colours of purple, pink, brown, and orange. The third one is a deep blue cotton hanker-chief style, which would be cool if the weather gets hot. That one could be really useful on holiday in the summer. I wonder if I will wear them and how I will feel? I am scared really – I think I will look so gaunt when I am bald as I am so long necked.

The Consultant Nurse suggested we made the task into a nice day so we took her advice and had a super lazy lunch at a country pub. Real quality time; which shows us what our retirement may be like in the future.

At bedtime I shed a few tears. I'm not sure if I like the wig now and I so want to feel and look good, and above all look 'normal'. Andy is understandably exasperated with me because no matter what he says it doesn't ease my anxiety about it all at the moment.

New stunning look

Thursday 8th March

Whilst Andy is at work I try the wig on, and fiddle with it to try and make it my own. It is beginning to appeal to me, but I still feel it is long and feels as though it needs a good cut. It is so different from my current hair in its' lank state. This is just something else to have to cope with and manage in order to look normal.

Friday 9th March

Hopefully this is the final visit about surgery. Today I need to have the stitches removed from the one and half inch wound and half-inch vein wound as well. I can't wait to get the dressings off and have a decent bath rather than a wash whilst sitting in the bath water. We see a different Consultant Nurse who removes the stitches. She is calm, sweet and supportive, and tells me about her own personal fight with the disease and past surgery. She is an inspirational and brave lady. Andy came with me as usual and is still supportive, positive and strong. I so love him.

I wore my wig today for two hours and I am beginning to like it. It is hot on top of my own hair, but I need to get used to my new look. It is especially strange when I walk past a mirror in the house and see the new me. This is going to be a huge jump into the unknown to have confidence and feel good about myself when wearing a wig in public.

Saturday 10th March

I decide to visit the garden centre for a birthday present for my niece Sarah and also to go out in public for the first time in my wig. It is a very strange feeling because I know I look different. It was an interesting experience as I thought everyone would look at me and know it was a wig but they don't, as I obviously look perfectly normal. A very odd feeling to say the least, but it has boosted my confidence a bit. There is still a long way to go though. Andy loves my wig and is constantly trying to convince me it is beautiful. He is very positive and knows this is very hard for me.

Sunday 11th March

I am feeling happier about my wig and today will be a new adventure. Karon and Andy have agreed for us to go to their house (with Chloe as usual) and then Karon is going to the opticians with me. I am due for an eye test and want a new modern look to cheer me up. I really fancy gold rectangular frames and a second pair with pink or purple frames. Currently I wear gold oval shaped frames all day, as they are vari-focal lens and I can't actually function without them, especially when reading.

I make the decision to wear my wig, so that I can plan the new look for the next few months, as I will be wearing the wig for at least that length of time. This would help raise my self-esteem and confidence if I knew I looked my best during the treatment. I am quite nervous when I walk into Andy and Karon's house but Karon (who is so close and honest and the very best friend you could have) instantly tells me how stunning and glamorous it is. I hope it doesn't turn heads too much! I don't want too much attention. I can't win really.

I end up buying four pairs of glasses and spending loads of money. I do now have fun, glamorous and everyday frames so they should cheer me up. We chill out over a lazy Sunday lunch. We visit Bella and Lee next door before we leave and they too are amazed at the new look and how well I seem. We arrive home at seven o'clock.

Tuesday 13th March

My mouth and gums are sore even though I have returned to gently using the electric toothbrush instead of a hand brush, which was recommended by the oncology nurses. I am used to the electric toothbrush for cleaning my teeth. I now have a white bead at the back of my throat and it hurts a bit. I decide to ring the oncology nurse who advises me to use anti-bacterial mouthwash and see how it goes. I sent Andy a text message asking him to buy some for me on his way home from work.

Thursday 15th March

I felt a bit poorly yesterday and by teatime my legs ached and I had the shivers occasionally. My mouth was still sore and by bedtime it hurt to swallow.

I had a terrible night's sleep as my throat has gone so sore and it is really painful to swallow and drink. I feel so bad that I have to ring the nurse again. She asks me to go to the hospital for the doctor to examine me. I just about managed to get dressed and drive there – they took a throat swab and blood test to check my blood count. The doctor examined me and prescribed a week's supply of antibiotics.

I go to bed at 11.30am and feel absolutely terrible. Andy has telephoned me twice to check I am OK, as I know he is worried about me. I am still in bed when Andy gets home from work at 5.30pm. I can hardly swallow, ache all over and feel so ill. I only got out of bed twice to let Chloe into the garden and feed her. After two antibiotic tablets I begin to feel a little bit better in the early evening and get up for an hour to try and eat the first thing all day. Bob and Dot were going to come for tea but Andy has cancelled them.

Saturday 17th March

I have been amazed how quickly I became ill, but then the immune system is at its' lowest this week. Apparently Lee has also got this bug; so guess who gave it to me on Sunday! I am also surprised how quickly I recovered once the antibiotics took hold. I feel much better today and my throat is improving well. I still feel a bit tired, but I am pottering about at home and well on the road to recovery.

I noticed my hair is beginning to shed odd hairs in the bath and in the sink when I brush it. This is the start of the horrible side effect. I am still absolutely dreading it and even though I know it has to happen as part of 'the insurance policy' it is still frightening. It feels unladylike and a real worry as to how Andy will react to me when it has all gone. The Consultant Nurse explicitly said it would all go completely and not even remain thin!

Monday 19th March

Andy left at 5.15am to go to Birmingham airport to fly to Turin for work. I should be OK. I know he worries about me but he has a job to do. He is due back about eight o'clock tomorrow evening so it isn't that long really.

My hair is now coming out in clumps if I pull it, and leaving loads in the bath too. It is strangely a very conciliatory moment when you flush the clumps down the toilet – one of those awful moments in life – most surreal, and very sad indeed. I can't somehow shed a tear but I do grit my teeth, which is a sign of stress for me.

I try to keep myself busy and wear my wig most of the day now – I have got used to it and the new style does suit me. I bought a wig stand when we bought the shampoo and conditioner. It is plastic and just two interlocking head-shaped pieces of plastic so it isn't very fancy. I leave it by the bed and drape the wig over it when I am not wearing it. The wig is amazingly easy to wash. I have followed the instructions and washed it by hand in lukewarm water with the recommended shampoo. Then I rinse it, shake it dry, and drape it over the stand. If I do it just before I go to bed it is dry by morning. As it is acrylic you can shake it and brush it and then it is back in the style as the acrylic has been heat set to remain that way. I will only need to do this about once a week. It is actually a lot less trouble than real hair in that aspect. I would rather have my own hair though.

I went to a supermarket to do a bit of shopping and to a home furnishings store to get some wall-paper samples for the bathroom – long way off that stage in the renovation yet! Andy rang me this evening, and Dad and Joyce my mother-in-law did too. They are all checking I am OK. Karon sends me texts most days, which is lovely.

Tuesday 20th March

My hair has really come out today and it is now down to a few wisps only. It looks horrible and without the wig you can definitely tell I am having chemotherapy treatment. It is a good job the wig looks very natural and everyone thinks it suits me and is stunning! I've never been called stunning before. I am also so determined not to look like a cancer patient if I can avoid doing so. I have started to wear a scarf whenever I leave the bedroom without my wig, as I do not want anyone to see me bald – even through the window.

Andy's flights are on time and he arrives home at eight o'clock. Chloe is so pleased to see him and makes a big fuss. She has been lovely company and I even enjoy walking her now after the surgery. Andy has a bit of a cold and feels tired so we get an early night.

Wednesday 21st March

Andy is full of cold this morning and decides to take time off work. He is a bit miserable really – typical man!

I visit the doctor for a blood test for my thyroid problem as the Consultant at the local NHS hospital thinks one is due. The doctor took the sample from my left arm and didn't choose to use the access device to my blood stream as he thinks that might complicate things for me. After lunch I also visit the private hospital for my blood tests ready for chemotherapy tomorrow. The Oncology Nurse uses the device to take the sample from, which is no more painful than the usual needle insertion from a syringe. The appointment is very quick and efficient – as usual with the private health care we are receiving.

Andy is much weaker by the end of the day and takes to his bed with aching limbs and the shivers. I think I must have passed it onto him from last week.

Thursday 22nd March

I arrive at hospital at 7.30am for my dose of chemotherapy. It is 8.40am when I have my consultation with the Oncologist. He is very thorough and asks lots of questions. He adjusts the medication to prevent heartburn and my eyes from being runny at night. It is ten o'clock when the Nurse calls me for the chemo drugs – it takes nearly half an hour to pump them into me. It was painful when she inserted the needle as the area was bruised from the blood tests yesterday. The waiting lounge is very pleasant and the positive aspect of waiting is being able to talk to patients and find out what the treatment entails for those several sessions ahead of me. I learn quite a lot really from snippets of information, which is reassuring and good preparation for the journey ahead.

I still feel very positive, strong, and capable of getting through this. Both of the Oncology Nurses comment on my positive attitude and how it will help me to cope with it all. They are delighted with my wig and new look. I didn't feel particularly strange in the waiting room with my wig on. Some patients have very little hair as they are emerging from the treatment or are wearing scarves during treatment.

When I get home Andy is still in bed feeling really poorly. He gets a phone call from his boss saying they are going to promote him two grades and increase his salary. I am delighted for him – it all means more savings and brings early retirement even closer!

Saturday 24th March

I feel OK today. A little tired but absolutely fine. I keep taking all the pills – thyroid, glucosamine for my joint problems, anti-sickness, antacid, steroids, and eye drops too. I have word processed a chart to track taking them, as some are taken once, twice, three, or four times a day and it certainly takes some following.

Dad and Joyce arrived at 11.30am and left at 6.00pm after having lunch and a light tea with us. I am tired when they leave as they love chatting and it is hard to keep up at times. They are really impressed with my wig and Joyce is very surprised as to how good and natural it looks. Dad appears impressed and less worried about me as he can see how well I am doing and how positive I am too. He talks about Mum quite a lot and compares my treatment to hers. She had a very natural looking wig too.

Sunday 25th March

I potter about today and do some household chores. I felt really well until about five o'clock when I went very tired and had an early bath and night – I was in bed for eight o'clock. It must be the chemo effects and all the chatter from yesterday! I had heartburn in the night and took two spoonfuls of a heartburn liquid which relieves the symptoms of gastro-oesophageal reflux. I have been fine since, which is really good news. The eye drops have also stopped my eyes from being runny at night.

Monday 26th March

Today I went to collect my new glasses (two of the four pairs). They seem really modern in style, especially the trendy designer label crimson pink and black frames. Andy likes them too. The lens seem weird in the gold framed set as the vari-focal lens have been changed and they will take a bit of getting used to in the next few days. It was really nice to spend some time shopping for new bras, tops, and a cardigan. It makes me feel better and I am trying to keep up-to-date and well dressed to continue to help me feel good about myself, especially whilst wearing the wig.

Wednesday 28th March

I am officially signed off from work today but as Jack

can't meet me I am going into work tomorrow. Rebecca has emailed me and wants to meet me for a coffee to welcome me back – not sure it can happen tomorrow but she is very supportive. She has been emailing me regularly and thinks I have handled myself with great dignity in extremely difficult circumstances. People's perceptions and opinions are surprising because I think I am doing what I should be – staying positive, strong, and focussed. Maybe not everyone does this.

I took myself to the wig shop, as my wig has become very loose on the crown now that most of my hair has gone except for the few wisps left. The assistant stitches it for me in the private room and I wear the scarf I'd taken with me to make me feel better whilst in there. I still don't like looking at myself without hair and no one other than Andy seeing me. It is just so horrible to deal with and so unladylike when you look nearly bald.

Bob and Dot came for tea and they are amazed at my wig. They think it is fabulous, and makes me look ten years younger. Dot wants one too! They really cheer me up with these comments. This is an unexpected outcome as I didn't realise I am beginning to change people's perceptions and expectations of cancer treatment. Jack rings me to give me an option about going into work tomorrow as he is recovering from a cold and is kindly thinking about my low immune system. We agree to keep our distance as I feel I need to break the ice and go in to see colleagues before the Easter break.

Thursday 29th March

I am really quite apprehensive as I drive to work. I haven't seen most people for two months and they haven't seen me with my hair longer and in a new style. I am greeted with such enthusiasm. They are all amazed as to how well I look. My skin is very clear (must be all the water), my hair (wig) is fabulous, my new gold-framed rectangle shaped glasses are modern and I constantly smile too - which seems to make a difference. I am beginning to realise that people expect you to look really ill and an obvious chemotherapy patient.

They love my hair. I just say 'thank you' and decide not to tell them that it is a wig. I only tell Paul who is a colleague and now my new line manager as part of the internal restructuring within the Service. He said it had never occurred to him and it looks so natural. That cheered me up immensely. I just keep saying to colleagues that it was my new look, new glasses, and a result of too much time to spend on beauty treatments.

Paul and I initially discuss the main projects and aspects of the work I could focus upon and how it could be more office based rather than school visit based to help to protect my immune system. They are all kind and supportive and just want to fit in with my plans and what I can offer them. It is quite emotional really as I am amazed and feel very humble as to how people are pleased to see me and keen for me to be back and yet concerned as to how I have been and what I have been through too. I am tired when I get home after three hours there, but once I have a rest I take Chloe for a short walk.

Andy and I agree it would be better to cut or shave the wisps of hair that are left, so that I look completely bald and clean-shaven. He gets the comb and scissors, but I end up in floods of tears, as I just can't let him do it. It feels like I am getting rid of the last part of me. I'll have to work up to it! This is an awful time in the treatment.

Saturday 31st March

I am still finding it hard to cope with my hair and can't cut the wisps yet at all. I want to but just can't do it. It is so personal and the baldness really is the worst part of the chemo. It is a good job I am happy with my wig, otherwise it would take a tremendous amount of coping with on a daily basis.

We enjoyed a relaxing pub meal with Andy and Karon last night. It was lovely to see them and we all enjoyed the chat. Karon still texts me most days: to touch base and keep my spirits up. I've tried some light gardening this week but it is so frustrating. I have to watch my back anyway and now can't push or pull with my right arm due to the lymph nodes having been removed. Just my luck to be right handed. I end up pottering and snipping, brushing up a bit, and cutting the dead flower heads off the daffodils. At least it will save Andy some time and I enjoy the fresh air.

Andy and I spent a lovely evening listening to a classical music concert. The meal afterwards was gorgeous and even though it was 11.30pm when we got home (which is really a late night for me now) it was worth it.

Monday 2nd April

I went into the bathroom after Andy had gone to work and doggedly gritted my teeth and cut my wispy hair. It was so hard but I managed not to cry, as I knew I would look terrible for the rest of the day if I did. I then shaved it quite short in an uneven sort of way, and hated the completely bald look. It is absolutely awful when you wash your face in the sink and lift your head up to dry it with the towel and then you see yourself in the mirror. I hate it. It also feels so cold – I really miss the warmth of hair. I sent Andy a text message.

'Have done the deed; please think of me as a baby hedgehog and not a bald wife.'

He replies: 'I knew it was only a matter of time!'

When he gets home I show him how I look without my wig. He swears he isn't turned off me and he thinks of it as 'only temporary.' I really hope it doesn't turn him off me, as I definitely don't feel beautiful or attractive without my saviour of a wig.

The 'Wow' Look

Wednesday 4th April

I am feeling well this week, which I am really pleased about, as my immune system is supposed to be low during these few days of the cycle. As I was so poorly with the throat infection last time I really want to stay well, so that I don't feel as though I am going to be ill every three weeks.

I took myself to the garden centre today to buy lots of vegetable seeds to plant on the patch we have in the garden. I feel positive about physically looking after it – once Andy has dug it over. I'll have to nag him to do that bit of hard work because I just can't do it, which is so frustrating. Mo my neighbour came round for a coffee again and a chat about my treatment, which is really helpful.

I am slowly getting used to the very close shaved head

look but can't say I am happy about it. I know everyone loves my wig. I am so pleased that I have made the conscious decision to wear a wig in public rather than scarves or hats. However, I would rather have my own hair. My underarm hair has also stopped growing – that's a positive! I don't seem to need to pluck my eyebrows as often either as they have obviously been thinning.

Saturday 7th April

We leave home in the morning to drive to Nantwich in Cheshire to leave Chloe for three nights with my mother-in-law Joyce. It is Chloe's second home and she is fine there. Andy and I drive to Conwy in North Wales for a three-night break in a hotel. The hotel and room are lovely and after a wander around we get freshened up, and have a wonderful dinner in the restaurant. We end up drinking too much and feel absolutely full from the food, but it is quality time together which is so lovely and important to us.

Tuesday 10th April

We had a really good time in Wales. It has given Andy and I a chance to reflect, chat, and scheme and plan for the future. I still feel very positive and strong and he is too, as well as being totally supportive. We still sometimes wonder just what the future will bring, even though the outcome looks curably. Only the years passing will prove that to be the case.

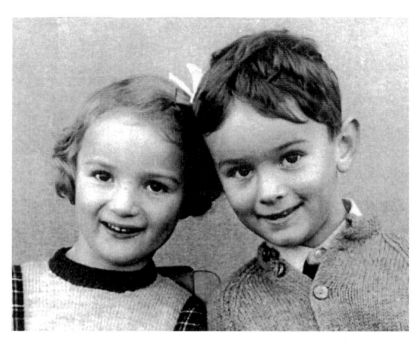

The Twins Alan and Susan

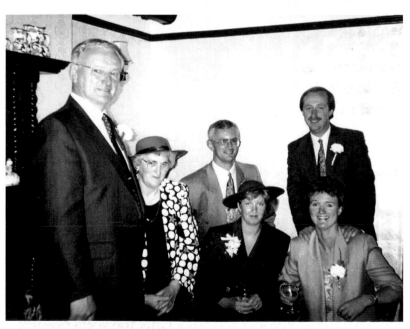

Dad, Mum, Alan, Gill, Andy & Sue 1994

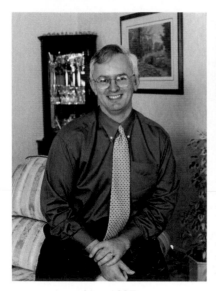

Alan 1997

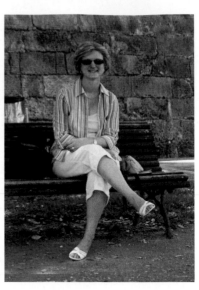

The wig Menorca 2007

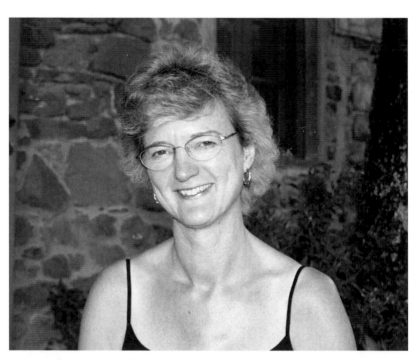

Summer 2006 Before Cancer

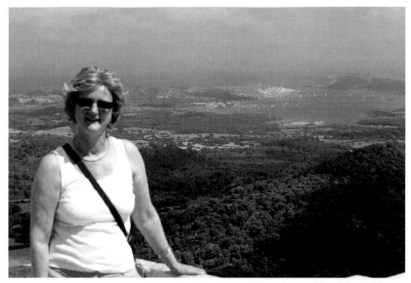

The wig Menorca 2007

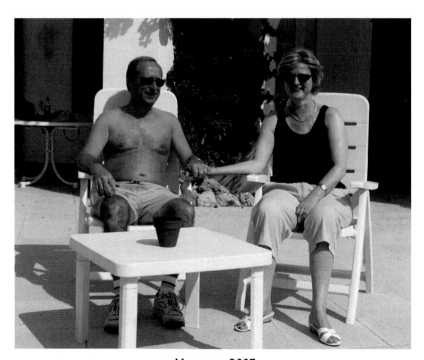

Menorca 2007

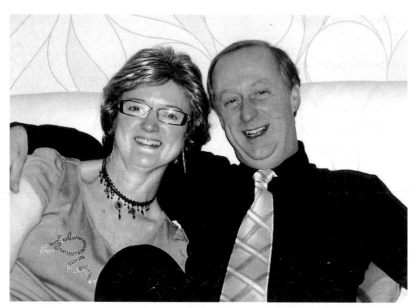

Pink & Black Party December 2007

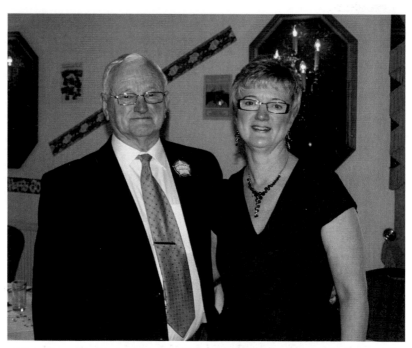

Dad's 80th Birthday October 2008

iv

We leave Conwy after another cooked breakfast and then meet my Auntie Margaret (Mum's sister), Uncle Brian, and Dad for lunch at a pub in Cheshire. Auntie Margaret is always very caring and supportive, and regularly telephones me. We also kept in touch when Mum was very ill and dying. Dad seems fine and chats away. He is obviously less worried about me now as I am keeping so well whilst on the chemotherapy.

I telephoned the opticians to stop them making up the other two pairs of glasses as I just can't get on with the gold framed pair, which I have had a couple of weeks now. I need to go in and see them about the problem.

Wednesday 11th April

I am very tired today after the few days away, not sleeping well in the hotel bed, too many hot flushes (which regularly wake me up), and all the travelling yesterday. I have a quiet morning pottering and then go to hospital for my blood test prior to chemotherapy tomorrow. I use the anaesthetic cream prior to going, in order to numb the area around my implant device, as it was so painful when they inserted the needle last time. This was due to bruising from the blood tests the day before. It is numb when they take the blood test and the Oncology Nurse puts an adhesive strip on it to stop the speck of blood from seeping onto my bra.

Thursday 12th April

It is an early start to be at hospital at 7.30am again for my third chemo dose. Time is flying really. I have an allergic reaction to the adhesive strip and the area is all red this morning. I use the anaesthetic cream again and the insertion of the chemo needle is fine. The nurse shows me the size of the needle – wow! It is bigger than a tapestry needle and no wonder they need good veins to insert it! The Oncologist seems pleased with my progress and state of health. He also agrees I can return to work on a part time and phased basis, which I am planning to do from Monday.

It is good to see the other patients and chat to them but it is 11.30am when I get home so it is a tiring morning. I feel fine otherwise and take the numerous pills during the day as instructed.

Friday 13th April

I visited the opticians today. They discovered they had put the wrong lens in my new gold-framed glasses. They have to keep them for a week to correct the problem. I have started to wear my designer ones. They are a raspberry pink with red, yellow, and black fine stripes along the arms. I can't cope without glasses and wear them all day. I was planning to wear this very modern pair for evenings rather than everyday but I now have no choice, as they are the only new pair I have at the moment.

Saturday 14th April

I have felt fine from the chemo treatment except this time I have felt a bit sickly off and on. I haven't been sick and I have no intention of doing so either! We went to Wendy and Clive's house for a meal in the evening, which was a great evening with friends. They think my glasses are stunning, which cheers me up immensely. They certainly give me a transformed, modern look with my new longer highlighted hairstyle.

Sunday 15th April

I am a bit constipated from all the pills (especially the steroids) and take a couple of sachets, which fortunately solves the problem. It is a lovely sunny day and we enjoy a cup of coffee at Joy and Peter's house for a couple of hours. It is good to see them and catch up with any news. Joy also loves my new stylish look and says she is surprised how well I look. Again, I think people just expect you to look ill and aren't sure what to expect when they see you.

Monday 16th April

I have been to work today for four and half-hours. It was still a bit nerve racking and I spent quite a lot of time chatting to colleagues who were pleased to see me. I had to keep repeating the story about my phased, part time return to work, and my new 'Wow' glasses and hairstyle. I didn't tell colleagues my hair is a wig. I feel I don't want that spread around the building and didn't want to spoil their illusions. I think if they have any family going through chemotherapy they would probably guess or wonder if it was a wig but didn't like to ask, so I didn't explain either. I just said 'Thank you' when they said how stunning and lovely the new hairstyle was.

I am still having lots of hot flushes and sweats, day and night. I was awake eight times last night, which is so disturbing and along with the hair loss is the worst part of all of this treatment.

Monday 16th April

I have returned from my third and last session in work this week. It has gone well but my brain hurts and I am quite tired in the evening. I was very tired last night and went to bed at eight o'clock. I feel less tired tonight. Andy reminded me that I was very tired on the Tuesday after the chemo last time. It could be that and not necessarily tiredness from going to work.

I was also constipated again for a couple of days, which is a side effect of the steroids that I have to take for three days after chemo treatment. I took a couple of the sachets again and it solved the problem. I only had heartburn once on Sunday, which is much better this time. My eyes are better overall and less runny but some nights they are worse again. I am still using the eye drops four times a day. The number of pills for the first week is amazing (24 for 3 days and 12 for 4 days) but they do control those potentially awful side effects so they are worth taking. All of the symptoms are manageable, but they are very wearing and make you feel unwell but not really ill. A lot of people wouldn't realise that I have to cope with these ailments, which may sound very trivial to some people, but all together they add up.

Sunday 22nd April

Andy and I went to a classical music concert again last night. It was a pleasant concert but not my favourite (too much soprano singing). We decided to eat at home rather than go out for a meal so that we weren't too late for me and I therefore wouldn't be so tired. He is also working very hard to juggle gardening and completing the refurbishment of the bathroom in his spare time.

We met Dad and Joyce for lunch at a pub in Staffordshire, as this is half-way for both of us. It was good to see them and chat, and also less tiring for me than travelling to Nantwich for the whole day. Dad seems OK generally and feels well supported by Edith his companion and friend. He started seeing her just at the same time as I was diagnosed, which I admit was difficult timing for me to 'get my head' around, but obviously positive support and company for Dad which is important. He looks well and more relaxed now that he knows I am doing well and looking good. He is being very strong and positive. He has coped very well so far with the impact on his family and better than I thought he would. I have also amazed myself as to how I have coped and how strong I have been after my absolute fear in January.

Tuesday 24th April

I have been to work yesterday and today, and I am tired this evening. I am enjoying being back at work, but it is mentally very demanding, especially when I have to recall information that I haven't specifically used since January. It is like dragging the details from the depths of my memory. Everyone is still so concerned about me and constantly keeping their eyes on me to make sure I don't overdo it. It will take me a few weeks to settle back and to find the level I can cope with alongside the chemotherapy and all the side effects.

Andy and Karon came for tea last night and we cooked gammon and chips, so it was easy to prepare. Karon is keeping her eye on me too and is a tremendous support – she still texts me everyday! She is very strong and bolsters my spirits if I show any signs of wavering at all.

Wednesday 25th April

I went to Lillian's house for lunch today – 'ladies that lunch!' It is really strange being able to do this, as I have never had the chance in my whole 31 years of full-time working. We had a great chat and she spoilt me with a three-course lunch. I don't think I need much tea this evening.

Thursday 26th April

I attended three quarters of a teaching and learning conference today. I left at 1.30pm and came home, as I was tired and needed to rest. It was rather daunting, as it was the first time I had seen some of the secondary Headteachers and school staff since my illness. They were all pleased to see me, asking how I was going on and how my return to work was going. I think many were surprised to see me at work whilst undergoing chemotherapy treatment and only two and half months after diagnosis. Jack realised it was a bit daunting for me, as he commented upon it as perhaps being an ordeal for me – he is still very supportive.

Bob and Dot came for a drink in the evening and left at ten o'clock, which was a bit late for me. I tumbled into bed extremely tired whilst Andy locked up.

Saturday 28th April

At eleven o'clock this morning the doorbell rang – it was the florist with the most stunning bouquet of flowers. They are yellow and red roses, and gerberas in silver paper. I couldn't work out who would send them to me. The card read: *"Missing you at the conference, get well soon from the Regional group."* I ended up in floods of tears, as these are other Advisers and Inspectors from across other Local Authorities who I know really well. I attend the termly regional network meetings to keep up-to-date. I have also attended the annual three-day conference, which requires staying away from home for two nights each year. I usually really enjoy it, feel the group members are friends, and keep up-to-date as a result, which helps me in my role. They are so thoughtful and unbelievably kind people.

Wednesday 2nd May

Work is going OK, although it is taking a while to get up to speed with all of the latest developments. I had a cup of coffee with Rebecca the Head of Service today. She was absolutely amazed at how well I looked and how strong I have been throughout this trauma. She is very supportive and caring and wants me to do what ever I think I can manage at work. They seem to greatly value my expertise.

I attended the Regional ICT meeting today. Rachel and Carl (ICT Consultants) also attended for the day. It seemed really strange networking, trying to feel up-to-date and full of enthusiasm. It is hard wearing a wig when most people don't know. It is something to handle and think about all of the time, as well as trying to be so positive about my illness. It does give me so much confidence though and I don't think I could walk into the room with a scarf or hat on instead.

I had to leave after lunch to drive to hospital for my blood test between 2.00pm and 3.00pm, ready for chemotherapy tomorrow. The treatment regime never goes away and so impacts on any sort of normal life. I feel as if I can't do anything completely or in its' entirety due to the treatment, tiredness, surgery impact, or tablet pattern.

Thursday 3rd May

It is the day of my third session of chemotherapy. Time is going very quickly and I remain totally committed to beating this *'bugger'* of a disease. I am very strong and positive, and cope by *'blinkering'* out what has happened to Alan and Mum. If I decided I was not going to survive I would give up now, so *'blinkering'* is my strategy to cope and remain focussed. I don't care what anyone thinks, but it is how I have chosen to deal with it and to climb Mount Everest in front of me. As the nurses have said, 'there is no right or wrong way to getting through this treatment.'

The Oncologist is very pleased with me at his consultation and the treatment goes well.

Friday 4th May

I have been into work today from 11.30am to attend some key meetings from 1.15pm to 4.30pm. On reflection, I don't think I should have done the block of time or at least I should have come home earlier as I am so very tired now.

The problem is that we were due to have a 15-minute break at three o'clock, but got two minutes only and then the meeting didn't finish until 4.50pm. I eventually got home at 5.45pm and therefore was out of the house for seven hours, which is too long for me, especially when I am full of drugs. I am gradually finding my own level of stamina and concentration, which is good, but also frustrating compared with the hours I used to work.

Sunday 6th May

Karon and Bella planned an *East Meets West* food buffet in my honour and to make sure I am still eating well. Fortunately I haven't lost my taste or appetite whilst on chemo. The food is fabulous and I definitely over eat on Bella's home-made vegetable samosas. Bella is a real expert at authentic Indian food.

I went very tired by eight o'clock (we arrived at 4.30pm) but did enjoy the laugh during the horse racing game that Andy organised. They certainly know how to have fun and how to spoil people. They are such good friends. Along with Bob and Dot, everyone is supporting me, and Karon constantly encourages me and tells me how proud she is of my progress.

I am constipated again for 24 hours due to the steroid tablets. I have to resort to the sachets again, but they do work! I also had heartburn twice last night but that was also manageable. The side effects could be a lot worse.

Monday 7th May

It is a Bank Holiday today and we have a day off work. It is a good job as I am tired – more tired than I have ever been and can't put one foot in front of the other. I think it is the chemo plus everything I have been doing over the weekend. Maybe the chemo has an accumulative effect and the tiredness gets worse each time. I had one rest on the bed mid-afternoon but didn't do much all day and went to bed very early at 7.30pm. My vision seems blurred at times too when I get tired.

Wednesday 9th May

I feel much better today and my tiredness has gradually lessened since Monday. I worked yesterday and improved during the time in work. My eyes felt a bit blurred as I arrived at work, but soon settled down.

Saturday 12th May

I went to collect a skirt and jacket that I had on order. I am pleased with them – just need some sunshine now to wear the skirt with a white top. It was tiring but I limited the bits of shopping I needed to do and had a good rest when I got home. I then prepared a meal for Liz and Richard. It was good to see them, as we had postponed them visiting us twice during my surgery period. Liz had visited me in hospital but neither of them had seen me with my new look. They were impressed and thought I looked so well – which fortunately I do!

Making eyes or not?

Sunday 13th May

Andy is making progress with the bathroom refurbishment, although it is taking a lot of his spare time. We made the effort today to go and choose some tiles. He then spent the afternoon working out the design and the number of tiles we need to order.

I feel tired today but nothing like last weekend. Work is going OK really and I now know my limits and what I can manage. It is still hard juggling it and looking after myself. They say being on chemotherapy is a long haul and tough regime – they are right.

Thursday 17th May

I have worked three consecutive days this week and don't

know if it has contributed to me being so very tired today. I am also upset about my eyelashes. They have been thinning for a couple of weeks. It has taken me ages every morning to try and put mascara on what it left so that they look normal. There are now so few eyelashes that I have had to concede and not wear mascara anymore – I think I look tired without them and feel so underdressed too. My eyebrows have gone very thin too. They are other set backs and signs of being on chemo – more side effects to hate.

I was trying to tell Andy whilst he was watching television and as he wasn't listening I accused him of not caring. He went wild at me and we had such a row – I moaned about all my frustrations and had a bad evening in tears. He is wonderful and I know he cares. I just feel so done by, frustrated, unladylike, and fed up with the tough regime of it all. I don't know what I would do without him, as I love him so much, and he is so patient with me and puts up with all of the side effects of the chemo. They certainly do impact on your partner too.

Saturday 19th May

Dad and Joyce came down for the day today. It was nice to see them both and they seem to be coping well. Dad does drive me nuts with his constant repeating of 'How nice it is to have a companion to talk to,' i.e. Edith. I still find this strange, but I wouldn't mind so much if he didn't keep repeating it. I think, perhaps, it is some form of justification on his part. I just feel it is being thrust down my throat all the time. He also keeps repeating one particular sentence.

'I watched my Mother die of breast cancer, then my wife, I've lost a son and now Susan has it.'

I don't want to upset him by saying anything, but I hate being added to the sentence as if I am dying of cancer too! I am fighting this *'bugger'* and remaining extremely positive so the sentence doesn't really please me.

Thursday 24th May

I had my blood test yesterday ready for the first dose of Stage 2 chemotherapy drugs administered this morning. I am a bit apprehensive as to how well I will be and how I will react to the three new chemotherapy drugs in this regime. Two were given by injection, which only took about 15 minutes rather than 25 as before. Apparently they are anti metabolite drugs, which stop cancer cells from making and repairing DNA cells, which they need to grow and multiply. These drugs have nasty side effects, because they stop the growth of normal cells in our bodies too, during the treatment. The third drug is in tablet form and is to be taken three times a day for two weeks – more pills to add to the chart!

The Oncologist was really pleased with my progress and how well I am doing – that gave me a boost. I drank a pint of Irish stout on Tuesday evening whilst doing the online food shopping. This was my way of boosting the red blood cells. He commented on how high my blood count was – even the nurse said it was very high. That is fine by me – along as there isn't any reason to delay my course of treatment it suits me fine – sooner done the better!

Saturday 26th May

I haven't been any worse with these drugs really. I felt very hot and fidgety during Thursday night, which resulted in a restless night (in addition to my numerous hot flushes). During Friday morning I looked very red and flushed in the face but it passed off during the day. I have to take six tablets from Friday morning until Saturday lunchtime, to help clear the toxins from my body, so maybe it was an effect of those. The drug is a derivative of folic acid and is used to prevent toxicity, following each treatment of the anti-cancer drugs.

I haven't felt sick at all. I had heartburn a bit this morning but it was sorted with a couple of doses of liquid. Constipation is an issue for these 48 hours so I am taking the sachets prescribed to sort that out. It seems like one long pill taking session and is such a strain.

Monday 28th May

We have had a restful, quiet weekend and now it is Bank

Holiday. Andy is at home from work until Thursday and I am off for the week – not sure if it is leave, sickness time or what – don't really worry about logistics anymore anyway. Andy is trying to spend his time finishing the bathroom and doing some gardening – those weeds will keep growing!

Thursday 31st May

I have had my second dose of the Stage 2 chemotherapy today. It was an early start at 7.30am at the hospital as usual. I saw the Oncologist who is pleased again and got in the car at 9.20am after the treatment. At least it gives me a chance to rest when I get home.

Friday 1st June

I look really red and flushed in the cheeks again this morning and feel a bit tired but not really ill. The redness does fade as the day progresses and I am now convinced it is the result of taking the six anti-cancer toxin tablets over the next 24 hours.

Saturday 2nd June

I don't feel too bad today after the chemotherapy – just a bit tired. I do feel my digestive system is a bit vulnerable, especially if I have a large meal and too much wine!

We have tickets for a concert at Symphony Hall and decide to go into our favourite restaurant after the concert. As long as I don't eat too much to make me feel uncomfortable and we are not too late, then I should be all right – ten o'clock is the latest bedtime for me really nowadays. My wig does enable me to go out and about and to socialise a lot really, as the world in general think I am normal and have absolutely no idea that I am going through chemotherapy.

Thursday 7th June

My hair is starting to grow back a tiny bit. It is slowly becoming less prickly and softer. It is such a relief that it will grow again. My eyebrows are growing quickly too and defining the lines with eyebrow-liner helps disguise the half grown look.

Saturday 9th June

I have been quite well all week – a bit tired, but probably not as much as on Stage 1 of chemotherapy. The constipation only lasted two to three days and was solved with the sachets. I only had heartburn twice, which again was quickly sorted with the favourite liquid. The hot flushes are still a real problem during the day and night. I get so hot and sweat so much under the wig when they happen during the daytime. I also go lobster red in the face so it is rather obvious – especially when I am at work.

We were due at Barry and Lillian's house tonight for a meal, but Barry is unwell so they have postponed it – everyone is kind in protecting me from infection. Andy and I ate in and enjoyed a bottle of champagne to celebrate the bathroom refurbishment being completed. He has worked hard to make such a beautiful luxury bathroom. It was a wonderful relaxing chill-out evening – what we both needed really.

The vegetable garden has been fun during the last few weeks. I have to work in it for short spells at any one time, because of my energy levels and back problems too. I really enjoy being in the fresh air and being busy. We have lots of salad ingredients, runner beans, courgettes and carrots coming to fruition. The fresh produce is helping to keep me fit and healthy.

Wednesday 13th June

A busy three weeks at work with an annual exhibition and Awards Ceremony to organise for over two hundred GCSE and A level Design and Technology students' work from most secondary schools in the Local Authority. It is a wonderful celebration of their work with the Rotary Clubs and many local companies involved. Next week will be very busy with setting up on Monday, judging the awards and prizes most of Tuesday, and the Awards Ceremony on Thursday evening (after chemotherapy in the morning). I so hope I am well enough to do the event.

Sunday 17th June

We had a busy weekend seeing friends and travelling to Nantwich in Cheshire today as it is Father's Day. Last night we enjoyed a super buffet meal for a few hours with Bob and Dot, Andy and Karon. They are great supportive friends who give me lots of encouragement.

Today we travelled up the M6 motorway (with Chloe in the back of the car) to Nantwich. We went to Joyce's for coffee and left Chloe there whilst the three of us went out for lunch to meet my Dad and Edith, his companion. She is really nice, with a good sense of humour, and I can see they both enjoy each other's company. Dad is still occasionally repeating how nice it is to have company. I am slowing getting used to the idea of Dad and Edith but think of Mum a lot. I was very tired when we got home at six o'clock after leaving at ten o'clock this morning. It was worth it though as it was good to see everyone and it was the first time we had visited Nantwich since early January because of my illness and treatment.

Tuesday 19th June

A very busy day today as I worked from 8.15am until 4.00pm which is longer than my usual five to six hours. It was worth it in order to be ready for the Awards Ceremony on Thursday evening and also not to be in work tomorrow - a day of rest! Judging of the students' projects (after setting up yesterday) and then completion of the certificates, prize cheques, photographs of winning projects, and the final arrangements made it very busy. The students have worked hard and this is a true celebration of all their work for GCSE and A level.

Thursday 21st June

My seventh dose out of twelve of chemotherapy today – we are getting there and I can see the end of this section of Mount Everest. The Oncologist is really pleased again. I talked to him about all the hot flushes and sweats that I have and how disturbing and embarrassing they are when I go lobster red, etc. He prescribed a hormone (low dose) used to treat breast cancer or ovarian cancer and asked me to take it for the week and let him know how I am when I go for dose eight.

I am either mad, heroic or a brick, but I got dressed up and left home at 4.30pm after a restful afternoon. I greeted the invited guests and dignitaries for a tour of the exhibition and then we all went to the Awards Ceremony. It was attended by over four hundred and fifty students, parents and teachers, and was such a celebration. I have to read out all two hundred and eleven names for the certificates to be presented and fifty-two names for the winners to collect their awards. That is no mean task any year! Most people didn't know I had chemotherapy this morning or that I was ill at all and I am convinced that is down to my fabulous natural looking wig. A lot of the teachers and Rotarians, guests and immediate work colleagues who knew were very concerned for me. I was so proud of myself. Rebecca (Head of Service) was unable to attend, but so concerned when she knew what I was doing and sent me a good luck message.

I was extremely tired when I got home at ten o'clock – some of it was relief and also the effects of chemotherapy.

Friday 22nd June

I feel tired this morning but able to go to the exhibition for an hour to meet the innovation winners and the local journalist. It was well worth the effort.

It all caught up with me, but only tiredness not illness. I was asleep at 1.30pm, then walked Chloe at three o'clock, asleep again at four o'clock, woke up an hour or so later with a boost of energy and cooked tea, ate tea and was in bed at eight o'clock. No constipation or heartburn to worry about which is really good news.

Saturday 23rd June

We went to Barry and Lillian's for a lovely meal and catch up chat. Barry's sister has just died from cancer – she has battled several times over 18 years and started with breast cancer originally. The disease touches so many families.

A chink in my armour

Wednesday 27th June

I am getting a bit excited (or is it relief!) as my hair is definitely growing – it is softer, feels like down, and looks darker. Andy has started to call me Ducky. A long way to go yet as it is only about three or four millimetres at the moment. It could take until next spring to get it to be like my wig. Blood test this afternoon for dose eight tomorrow. Nearly over this hurdle in the journey up the mountain.

Mo rang me today to see if she could go with me to walk Chloe each day. She wants to lose some weight, but doesn't want to walk in the lanes by herself. It is good to have some company and also I can talk differently to her since she went through the same experience with breast cancer.

Thursday 28th June

Chemotherapy again today – dose eight – I am getting there and can see the end of the treatment (last dose is 23rd August). I talked to the Oncologist about the hot flushes and the fact the hormone tablets made me even redder and I feel as though I am boiling rather than just hot. He suggests I persevere with them for the next three weeks. I suppose it is worth a go, as the sage oil capsules I've been taking since March have made no difference at all.

We are due to fly to Menorca in four weeks time and I am so looking forward to spending some quality time with Andy in the villa and around the pool. I still feel pretty good, and although I do get tired, I have learnt to rest in between activities and listen to my body as advised by my Oncologist.

Sunday 1st July

We had a super relaxing meal and chat at Andy and Karon's last night. It was good to see 'my sister' and to catch up too.

Today we went to Roger and Kate's for a relaxing Sunday lunch. They were going to barbecue, but as usual hefty intermittent showers were forecast – and they arrived! The food was fabulous and the support of friends is amazing. They all help me to remain so positive, strong and determined. As I say to people, 'They say it is curable and I have to believe that until time proves it right or wrong'.

Monday 2nd July

I worked today from eleven o'clock until 4.30pm and arrived home at 4.50pm. As I felt reasonably OK I decided to get changed into my jeans and to take Chloe for a walk and then to rest afterwards. Mo wasn't at home to go with me so I carried on as Chloe needed to go out. Big mistake! I nearly didn't get home as my energy and stamina ran out about three hundred yards from home at the end of the 20-minute walk. I nearly sat on a stack of building blocks outside a neighbour's house to recover. Andy was home when I got back and I collapsed onto a kitchen stool, put my feet up, and did not move for 15 minutes – that was how long it took me to recover. Big lesson learnt – I should continue to rest for an hour when I get in from work before I take Chloe for a stroll. It is absolutely amazing how the chemotherapy drugs have now drained my stamina.

Wednesday 4th July

I suddenly realised today that I have not had a single hot flush or sweat all day. Considering I could have six to eight a day and at night it is fabulous – I hope it continues.

Sunday 8th July

Andy was collected at six thirty this morning to be driven to Heathrow airport to fly to India until Thursday night. He has agreed to go on a compact short trip in a week when I am not on chemotherapy – to suit him and me. I feel lost without him. I so love him and realise I depend upon him so much. I walk Chloe about eight o'clock and have a restful morning before going to Bob and Dot's for an annual birthday lunch with about 20 of their friends.

It is a super meal and great fun but because I arrived at two o'clock I decided that I needed to leave at about five o'clock – just before the quizzes and games start, and well before I get too tired. It is hard being there on my own and really hard to leave early. I try to exit quietly, but Bob teases me that I need to go for the dog, until I have to explain that it is for my health's sake. At which point a crack in my armour opens up and I end up crying as I leave. Dot is very concerned. Bob's comment was unintentional but shows how vulnerable I am at times. I ended up crying all the way home and most of the evening – even when Andy rang to say he was in the hotel in Mumbia. I was distraught and just couldn't stop crying – I felt so lonely, vulnerable, and realised how very hard it is to be positive, strong, and cheerful one hundred percent of the time.

Monday 9th July

I slept restlessly and felt dreadful in the morning. I got

up to see huge swollen eyes and not a pretty face at all. It took me most of two hours, including walking Chloe, to decide if I could: a) face colleagues at work; and b) cope with work; and c) make the effort at all.

I eventually made the decision to pull myself together, and sort out my make-up as best I could. I still have no real eyelashes to add mascara to, which would make my eyes appear much larger and more sparkling. One of the reasons for going to work was that it would be a long day and night at home on my own if I didn't. I managed it and was glad I made the effort. A lot of people really wouldn't have any idea how hard it is coping on a daily basis with all of this and pulling yourself together when you get really low and a chink is found in your armour plating.

Dot rang me to see if I was going on OK. She told me that some of her friends had absolutely no idea I was on chemotherapy when they told them after I had left. They were completely thrown by how well I looked, and the effect my wig had on my new modern look. I must confess it really cheered me up, as I know the wig is changing people's perceptions and expectations - if that is a good outcome of this treatment then it will be a bonus too.

Thursday 12th July

Andy arrives home at about nine o'clock tonight and I will be so pleased to see him. I really miss him, feel unsafe without him, and realise how much I need him and depend upon him too. He has had a really busy trip and his homeward journey is 20 hours travelling in total, which is exhausting.

I am tired, as I have had to take Chloe for a walk (even if it is a short one) in the mornings before work and in the afternoon after my rest. You also realise how much you do for each other such as locking up, topping up the bird feeders, and doing all the cooking and clearing away – instead of sharing the roles. I have managed and feel proud of myself, apart from getting so upset on Sunday.

Monday 16th July

We had a quiet weekend pottering about at home and doing a few chores. We were both tired after last week, so had early nights and lie-ins, which was lovely. It is good to spend time together, relax, chat, and appreciate each other. This year has really made us closer, stronger, and more in love than ever.

Tuesday 17th July

I worked this morning, but left the school at the start of a meeting and went back to the Office. I was due to meet with the Headteacher and two external consultants about future building plans. One of the consultants was full of cold, spluttering and coughing terribly. I decided that I needed to put myself first and avoid infections. I gave my excuses and left the meeting before it even started. I can't guarantee my immune system isn't low and therefore can't fight infection. I felt quite rude really, but knew I had to do it to protect myself.

Wednesday 18th July

I finished work for the week today as I had a blood test again this afternoon. It is dose nine out of twelve – time is going so quickly. Schools finish on Friday for the summer break, so I'll go in next week to sort out things and put my desk in order before the holiday to Menorca. We fly out on 27th July and I can't wait to spend time with Andy in the villa and by the pool.

A lovely meal with Bob and Dot, and Andy and Karon finished the day beautifully. It was a bit late to bed for me (11.00pm), as I get tired so easily, which is frustrating, and does inhibit normal activities. We are all off on holiday sometime next week so it was lovely to meet up before then.

Thursday 19th July

I got bitten on the arm yesterday afternoon as I returned from my daily walk with Chloe and Mo. I have no idea what it was but the Oncologist was rather concerned about the two and half inch wide red mark. He prescribed a hydrocortisone cream to use four times a day – more medication – to reduce the risk of infection.

My blood count was normal again so the chemotherapy was administered as usual. It was an OK morning with only one nurse on duty and there weren't too many of us this week. I arrived at 7.30am and left at 9.20am, as I was first to get the drugs today.

My hair is growing quite well and is about one centimetre long – I have no intention of going without my wig until it is about five centimetres long and restyled – that could well be October or November time. It is a long year! My eyebrows are more or less normal now and the eyelashes can just about take mascara if I chose to wear it. I feel much better about myself.

Saturday 21st July

Dad, mother-in-law Joyce, and Edith have been for the day. They arrived about 11.30am and had to drive through quite a few floods on parts of the roads near here – there had been torrential downpours yesterday.

We enjoyed them coming and I did a leg of lamb with vegetables, and made a summer pudding. I did some of the preparation on Friday, as I was at home and also to make Saturday less tiring for me. They do chatter non-stop, which is tiring in its own way, so I went on the bed and dozed for an hour to get some rest. Dad and Edith seem to enjoy each other's company and he didn't mention justifying it - except just once! He seems to be managing very well, and I am sure Edith has helped this as he has someone to talk to, when he is worried about my future. I was in bed at eight o'clock as I was very tired after they had left at 6.30pm.

Monday 23rd July

I went to work this morning for five hours to do a lot of sorting and clearing out as the Office is being re-organised to accommodate more colleagues from September. It was a good feeling to sort my resources out, as I haven't had chance all year due to being off sick for at least two of the holiday periods. The atmosphere is more relaxed when the schools are on holiday and we are still working. I always call it 'Me time.'

Wednesday 25th July

I managed to do all my clearing away at work by two o'clock yesterday, so I didn't need to go in this morning. Blood test again this afternoon for the second dose of the three of the four cycles in Stage 2. Only two more doses to go! I visited the chiropractor too to get my joints checked and unlocked to keep on top of my back and neck problems.

Thursday 26th July

My blood count was fine again. It was the longest morning ever... when I arrived at 7.30am the waiting lounge was packed and only one nurse was on duty. She was doing her very best. I eventually left at 11.40am!

It was 12.30pm when I got home given that I collected a posy of flowers for Andy to put on Mum's grave for us. He is driving to Nantwich to his Mum's later this afternoon to take Chloe for her stay whilst we are in Menorca. It will be two years on 2nd August since Mum died of breast cancer. What would she think of me having to battle the same disease, only 18 months after she died, but 20 years younger than her. Surely it has to be genetically linked as well as other factors.

Friday 27th July

I finished the packing this morning and we arrived at Birmingham airport at 1.30pm to check-in for our 3.15pm flight to Menorca. It all went smoothly and we collected the hire car with no queues, which is amazing.

The villa is wonderful. We have rented the lower floor (which is classed as a two-bedroom villa) of a huge house set in one-acre grounds. It is awesome, with terraces, a kidney shaped ten metre long swimming pool, a huge garden with palm trees, pots, statues, gravel driveway, and a balustrade terrace. There is a swing seat with a canopy, which will be fabulous for me to sit and read in the shade and also to do some cross-stitch embroidery.

It is a bit frustrating not being allowed to sunbathe because the skin is so sensitive and will burn quickly - one of many side effects of chemotherapy. There is more to life than a suntan so I'll be very sensible.

Monday 30th July

We had a quiet, chill weekend, doing the food shopping, barbecuing steak, unwinding in the pool and lazing in the shade. I was tired after the travel on Friday, combined with a long day after chemotherapy treatment the day before. All my medicines got through the airport security in the visible plastic bags you have to use nowadays.

We visited the lovely harbour of Formells today and wandered around a bit. I am so limited on stamina that we have to keep stopping, sitting, and going in the shade. I am wearing a striped shirt over my t-shirt and cropped trousers with plenty of suntan cream, so that I am well protected. We sat and had a wonderful three-course lunch and a couple of beers at a harbour-side restaurant. Unknown to me the starter was laced with strong garlic, which went straight through me with my delicate system. Fortunately we made it back to the villa in time before I was ill. I felt quite poorly really.

I decided that my wig may be very hot in the sun, especially when I am in the shade by the pool. Last week I bought a white Baker's boy style hat – like a flat cap really. When I tried it on in the shop I had to go into the fitting room to try it on because it had to fit without the wig, which is quite bulky. It is great for by the pool and when sitting or eating on the terrace. My very short down like hair just shows around the edges so it looks like I have a crew cut. This gave me a lot of confidence in case anyone saw me. When the holiday representative came to see us I wasn't worried, as she didn't know me anyway, and probably just thought I had very short hair with my new sun hat on – chemotherapy probably never crossed her mind!

Tuesday 31st July

I have been ill with diarrhoea three times in three hours this morning. My system is so painful and upset as a result of the different foods, strong garlic, and chemotherapy too. I had to take tablets to stop the problem and fortunately they did work.

We decided to eat in again, with light meals of roast chicken and white fish. Andy seems quite content, very patient, and happy to be at the villa. I feel very upset and frustrated that I am suffering and how it is restricting the holiday. The temperature is lovely – 28-30°C in the sun and 25°C in the shade with a fabulous warm breeze. Heaven - after all the rain in England before we left.

Thursday 2nd August

It is three years today since Mum died whilst we were on holiday in Florida. I remember it was one of the most difficult decisions of my life to leave with Andy and fly to Florida on the Friday. She had been admitted into the hospice on the Wednesday. She died on the Tuesday after we had arrived and I shall never forget her. I did feel for Andy, as we had to cut the holiday short by a week. He has had to put up with a lot over the years really.

This holiday is great apart from the sensitive tummy and having to be careful as to which foods I eat. My stamina level and tiredness are a bigger issue now than they were a few weeks ago. I seem to be able to walk around for about 15 minutes then I run out of energy and have to sit on a seat in the shade to recover for at least ten minutes. I can walk Chloe at home for 20 to 30 minutes each day, but I have a long rest before and afterwards, whereas touring around a resort and looking at the sights is another issue entirely. I just can't do much and today in Mahon it was a tremendous effort to get back to the car. We were about ten minutes walk from the car park. The good thing was a long lazy lunch by the harbour again to chill, eat, drink, and chat. At least we are not in a rush!

I tried to be extremely careful with the choice of food for lunch to avoid any strong garlic. I chose asparagus and prawns, but amazingly they were stir-fried in olive oil with at least three cloves of garlic. Needless to say I was rushing to the toilet with diarrhoea as soon as we got back to the villa. It does make me feel fed up and poorly.

Monday 6th August

Today is our thirtieth (pearl) wedding anniversary and we decided to go into Mahon to treat ourselves by purchasing a Swarowski crystal ornament as we did the same on our silver wedding day too. I have always wanted another budgerigar as a pet so we purchased an ornament of two budgies on a perch. I called the male Kevin (a long-standing joke) and jokingly said the girl would be Kylie. The names have stuck and they are now referred to as Kevin and Kylie.

I feel quite a lot better as regards my sensitive tummy, so we decided to celebrate at an English owned restaurant in the evening. It was a beautiful place and we thoroughly enjoyed the romantic meal together. We are so much closer as a result of the cancer trauma and Andy is very positive and supportive. He is a wonderful husband really.

Tuesday 7th August

Today is Andy's birthday so we had a wonderful lazy lunch at a gorgeous harbour side restaurant in Es Castell. The lunch was fabulous and the grilled fish was perfect.

The evening was relaxing at the villa and we opened a

bottle of champagne to celebrate our wedding anniversary and Andy's birthday. We then ate some cold chicken and salad, had some wine and liquors too. Probably not a very wise thing to do at all!

Wednesday 8th August

I am so frustrated with the chemotherapy and its' after effects on everyday life. I ended up with awful heartburn for two hours in the night — my own fault I suppose after all of the alcohol, but still a nuisance after a fabulous two days.

Thursday 9th August

The holiday has been so relaxing and the right sort of holiday for me this year. The villa has been stunning, clean and well equipped. Perfect for the extra time we spent in it as a result of my limitations.

I have enjoyed the quality time with Andy who looks tanned and relaxed. Reading and attempting cross-stitch embroidery, on the swing seat in the shade at 25°C with a fantastic breeze, has been fabulous.

Saturday 11th August

We had a long day yesterday and I am really tired today.

It is a day of washing and resting, with Andy mowing the lawn and tidying the garden.

The flight back from Menorca wasn't until 7.30pm so after we left the villa we had a lunch in the restaurant at Es Castell, which is only ten minutes away from the airport. It was ten o'clock when we got home so it was late for me, after a mixed day of rest and activity. The tiredness is definitely worse, even though I have been on holiday. It is obviously an accumulative effect of the chemotherapy.

Sunday 12th August

It has been an enjoyable but very long day. We went to Andy and Karon's for a coffee at eleven o'clock as we haven't seen them for a while. It was good to catch up about holidays.

We then left at one o'clock and drove to a village near Chester for my Auntie Margaret and Uncle Brian's golden wedding open house event. I am very close to Auntie Margaret, (Mum's sister) and we regularly telephone each other to chat. The event was beautiful and we saw Dad and Edith to chat to as well. It was great to see my other aunts and uncles and also many of my cousins and their families. They were all amazed how well I look and how I seem so positive during the treatment, even after what I have been through. I think they really did expect to see someone in a scarf or hat and not someone looking very normal in my fabulous wig.

It was very difficult to get away and we eventually left at 6.15pm and arrived at Joyce's house at 6.45pm to collect Chloe. She was very pleased to see us and looked well and happy, obviously having been well cared for. She and Joyce enjoyed the holiday together and Andy's brother, Graham, also walked her and enjoyed her company too. Unfortunately it all meant that by the time we had travelled back down the M6 motorway it was 9.30pm when we got home. A very long day indeed!

Wednesday 15th August

Today I am beginning to feel more myself after an awful two days of complete lack of stamina, energy, and being desperately tired. Sunday on top of Friday, on top of being on chemotherapy, have taken their toll!

I would not have been in work if I was due to (off this week anyway) as I couldn't put one foot in front of the other. This is the side that many colleagues, friends, and family don't see. Those who saw me on Sunday will have the very positive and healthy image of cancer treatment, whilst some days it just isn't like that. I think I have become strong and determined to be positive and lead as normal a life as possible, but it does take its toll on my health sometimes.

Thursday 16th August

It is dose eleven of twelve today and next week is the last dose – Alleluia!

My blood count is normal again and the chemo is administered without any problems. The Oncologist discussed radiotherapy, which is the next stage. I am disappointed really when he tells me I will have 22 consecutive sessions – I was hoping for 17 to 20 - but we might as well get it zapped at this stage so it doesn't come back.

I have been given an appointment for ten o'clock on Wednesday 29th August at the Queen Elizabeth Hospital, Edgebaston, Birmingham. I will attend as a private patient in the NHS hospital. This first appointment is for the simulator and planning session. The Oncologist also tells me he will try to arrange for my implant device to be surgically removed by the Consultant on the afternoon of the 29th. Could be a busy day! They certainly don't hang about with the cycle of treatment – we have no reason to complain about any of the medical treatment and care.

Tuesday 21st August

I am supposed to be working for three days this week (well part-time hours anyway), but the Office desk re-arrangements are not yet complete. I have chosen to work at home on some reading, sorting out and forward planning, which is easier than trying to go into the Office.

Wednesday 22nd August

I received the letter today to confirm the surgical removal of the implant device next Wednesday afternoon. That is two appointments in one day, so it will be a lot to cope with mentally, along with the lack of stamina and tiredness from chemotherapy due tomorrow.

I had my blood test as usual and then decided to go into town for a while to shop for some new clothes. I feel I won't get much opportunity once I am coping with work and daily radiotherapy appointments. I spent a while in one department store and purchased a suit (an on the spur of the moment buy) and a skirt. After about three-quarters of an hour shopping I walked to another store to look for a top to wear with the skirt. It was another huge mistake – my stamina dropped suddenly (like it does!) and I felt like an empty shell. I had to walk back to the car very slowly and was glad to sit down, rest and recover in the car before I could drive home. It is so frustrating and there is nothing you can do about it when the body suddenly feels as if *"it has run out of petrol."*

A milestone

Thursday 23rd August

Today is a real celebration as it is the final twelfth dose of chemotherapy and six months from the start on 1st March.

I was given priority treatment by the nurses and was in the car ready to drive home at 8.30am - an absolute record! It is a fabulous feeling and everyone says how well I have done, and how positive and strong I have been throughout the six months. I decided to be brave and ask the Oncologist for his view on the likelihood of the cancer returning. I have to confess that as I asked the question I thought, 'Do I want to hear the answer really.' He is very optimistic and said he thought the likelihood of the cancer returning was 10-15% (based upon statistics). There is a 10-40% risk of cancer occurring in the left-breast as there is a higher risk of that with lobular cancers. I was really pleased as no one can give you a guarantee it will never return. 10-15% is the best news for weeks. I rang Andy who was delighted too and said he would celebrate with a cup of tea at work as that is all he had!

We shared a bottle of champagne in the evening to celebrate such a stepping-stone and a really good prognosis for the future. I walked Chloe in the afternoon and Mo was delighted for me as well. I gave her a bunch of flowers for her birthday today and as a thank you for her support and friendship.

Saturday 25th August

We travelled to Nantwich mid-afternoon as we were invited to tea at Auntie Jen and Uncle Norman's house. Norman is my Mum's younger brother and has been supportive throughout and regularly telephones me.

We called for a cup of tea with Dad and to tell him my news. He seemed pleased, but I am not sure he realised what it really meant to me. I suppose other people don't know how you feel about this disease all of the time. We went to Joyce's house and left Chloe with her whilst we went out for the meal. It was lovely to spend time with Norman and Jen, and Andy and Karon, our friends too. (Andy is a younger brother of Jen – very complicated family links). We arrived home at 12.30am.

Sunday 26th August

My stamina levels are at zero today and I am extremely tired after yesterday. It was too long on a chemotherapy weekend. My tummy and system have also been very sensitive and I have ended up with diarrhoea again. We thought it was the change of food in Menorca four weeks ago, but obviously my system has taken such a battering with all the drugs for six months that it is now very delicate indeed.

Tuesday 28th August

My tummy is beginning to settle down today after three days of sensitivity and feeling quite ill at times. It has also taken me two days to get over our visit to Nantwich. You have to question whether it was worth it really, although I know it was and we are trying to keep in touch with family and friends throughout this horrendous period.

I am so fed up of not feeling fit, energetic, or really well. Everyone says how well I look (which I do), but they don't realise the ongoing ailments and side effects you are either controlling with medication (i.e. anti-sickness, ant-acid, heartburn solutions or diarrhoea tablets); or having to manage everyday and, above all, 'listen to the body'. It will be good to feel more energetic in a few months time.

I worked for four-and-half hours today, sorting myself out in the Office, as I won't be in for the rest of the week due to surgery. It is non-stop and relentless treatment, but

I do feel that I am slowly climbing Mount Everest. We are near the next stage now.

Wednesday 29th August

Today is a big, busy, complex day for me on top of a weekend of chemotherapy, and the ongoing reduced tiredness levels.

Andy has taken special leave from work to be able to take me to both hospital appointments. He hasn't been to an appointment with me for six months as I went to all the chemotherapy ones on my own. We agreed this was the best use of time and I could talk to other patients easier without him feeling bored or embarrassed. He is still wonderful, positive, supportive, and 'my rock'.

We have an appointment at the Queen Elizabeth Hospital, Edgebaston, Birmingham for ten o'clock, so will have to leave home at 8.50am to allow travel time. It is the main Cancer Centre in the West Midlands. I am then due into the private hospital, which is in a different direction, as a day patient for surgery to remove the implant device. It is a 15 to 20 minute operation and I will be home this evening.

Friday 31st August

I have been tired today as the after effects of the anaesthetic caught up with me. I have had a lazy sitting about day and was too tired to take Chloe for a walk, so Andy took her after work.

The visit to the Queen Elizabeth Hospital was an experience. There are three hospitals on one site, plus building work for a huge new hospital. Hence there are builders, machinery, temporary roads, pathways, and lots to negotiate. We managed to park and find the Cancer Centre just on time. The appointment lasted about 40 minutes. It was quite a weird experience lying on the bed being lasered, x-rayed, measured, and ink marked for precision. They have applied a permanent tattoo - two very small marks to enable them to line the machines up accurately each time. I don't really mind these marks being permanent - in case they need them again. I don't expect them to as far as I am concerned!

The operation in the afternoon was straight-forward and I was home for seven o'clock. Andy cooked rice and defrosted chill-con-carni, so it was easy and simple for us both. Chloe was glad to see me home and Andy believed she sensed something was different when he returned to walk her without me, whilst I was in the operating theatre.

My surgery area is a wonderful deep purple bruise all around the dressing area and extends about six to two inches (15 centimetres to 5 centimetres) left of my left breast – very colourful but not painful or sore, therefore manageable. I had to do some thinking prior to going in for the operation. I just didn't want to have to walk to theatre in my dressing gown and also bald. My way of dealing with the hair loss is to look normal when wearing my wig. I asked the nurse if I needed to remove my wig for surgery and much to my surprise she said I didn't. I had taken my Baker boy hat with me thinking, 'I could at least walk down the corridor wearing that instead of my wig.' Before you lie on the couch outside the theatre, you have to remove your dressing gown and slippers, and then the nurses tuck them into the base of your bed, so when the porters push the bed back after the operation they go back to your room too. It meant when I came around I was still wearing my wig and looking as regal as ever!

Saturday 1st September

It is exactly six months today since my first dose of chemotherapy and insertion of the device the day before. It seems a long time, yet it has gone surprisingly quickly too.

We had a lovely time last night as I managed to find the energy to go to a Sci-fi music theme concert at Symphony Hall. We had bought tickets for Andy (as in Andy and Karon), and for my Andy too, for both of their birthdays in August. It was a great concert and we enjoyed a meal out. It was an effort but I did manage it.

I was a bit upset that Dad hadn't telephoned to see how I was until today. I think that he just hadn't got the 29th

August events registered in his mind for some reason and so hadn't realised that I had been in hospital again. When I was talking to him on the phone he apologised once he was aware of the situation.

Monday 3rd September

I eventually perked up and felt more like myself yesterday. I have been to work today at 12 noon supposedly until 5.15pm, when a meeting was taking place. As usual it over ran until 5.30pm, so it was 6.10pm when I got home and I was absolutely mentally drained.

Andy walked Chloe. I cooked tea, ate tea, cleared away and was in bed at 8.30pm. Some of my colleagues think I am fantastic and look so well, but they don't realise how disciplined I have to be to rest and sleep to enable me to do the part-time work at all.

Just zap it

Wednesday 5th September

Today has been a big day and another milestone for me.
It is the next step up Mount Everest and marching
towards those Christmas lights at the top! I went to work
this morning for an hour-and-half to tie up some loose
ends and mainly to keep my mind occupied.

I went to see the Consultant at 12.15pm to have my
stitches removed from the surgery last week. He was very
pleased with my progress overall. He will take over from
the Oncologist at the end of the radiotherapy. I will then
have medical check-ups every three months until it is 18
months from diagnosis, which takes me to mid summer
next year. After that I will have six monthly checks until
it is five years from diagnosis, which is very reassuring.

Andy took me for my first radiotherapy treatment at the

Queen Elizabeth Hospital at 3.50pm. We had to wait a few minutes for treatment and it is a 50 or 60 minutes drive each way, as it is right through the middle of Birmingham and five miles the other side of the City centre. We have been given a paper pass to show the car park attendant and can park in the lower section of the multi-storey car park, which is only 30 metres from the Cancer Centre and free. This is really convenient compared with other patients having to find parking, pay for it, and then walk to the various centres as well. I must confess we are both impressed with this organisation for all radiotherapy patients whether NHS or private.

The radiographers work as a team of four. They have provided me with an appointment card, which I have to put in a tray outside the treatment room so they know I have arrived. The treatment room is one of eleven. Apparently they treat over three hundred patients each day. I have a gown in a brown paper bag in a numbered tray on a specific shelf in the waiting area. This means I can collect it each time, and change into this elegant dark green loose front popper gown, and then wait to be called in. The gown has poppers on the shoulders too so they can open the one side where treatment is required.

Thursday 6th September

I have to see the Oncologist at nine o'clock every Thursday morning at the private hospital, throughout the 22 days of radiotherapy. He is very pleased with me today. It is reassuring to be physically examined and checked every week. He always checks the neck, breasts, underarm areas, and liver for any signs of the disease. He has told me I am not allowed to use any soap on my right breast, nor antiperspirant on my underarm throughout the treatment, as this can encourage soreness. Even more rules and abnormal procedures to manage within my daily routine.

Radiotherapy is only two 30-second treatments and about a five minute appointment, whilst they line up the machinery with the two pinhead tattoos. Each visit the nursing staff greet me by asking me to confirm my name, date of birth, and first line of my address. It is reassuring to know they are making sure they have the correct patient. I have also noticed that the radiotherapy team constantly check with each other, as they set the measurements and double check all calculations. They disappear out of the room during the actual radiotherapy – safety from radiation I guess.

I think of Mum a lot, as I drove her from Nantwich to Christie's Hospital in Sale near Manchester on three occasions during her 15 days of radiotherapy. I can see her now as a tired lady walking slowly into the treatment room. I never thought that nearly four years later I would also be having regular radiotherapy visits.

Friday 7th September

The last few days have been extremely tiring as I have had six medical appointments in three consecutive days (three for radiotherapy with two to three hours of travel in the afternoons, stitches removed on Wednesday lunchtime, and Oncology check up on Thursday morning). The sixth appointment that I just had to fit in at 5.00pm today was to visit the chiropractor. I have had intermittent pain down my right leg for most of the week and I just knew that my back was not good. It turns out it is a disc irritating a nerve and a new problem for me. This is all I need at such a busy time. Matthew the chiropractor manipulated me and a fragile, gentle weekend was then the instruction.

I am so tired and fed-up with so much to cope with. Andy and I are doing fine really and taking a day at a time but it is an extremely long haul and very intense treatment period. I drove myself to radiotherapy, which gave Andy a break, and I gained a huge sense of achievement to drive through the underpasses in the middle of Birmingham and the return trip in the Friday rush hour traffic. I then drove another 20 minutes each way to the chiropractor appointment.

Monday 10th September

It has been lovely this weekend not to have to go to the Queen Elizabeth Hospital for treatment. Back again this afternoon for number four of 22!

Friends, Wendy and Clive, came for a meal on Saturday evening. It was great to see them and I managed to prepare a meal that didn't involve too much preparation. We met Dad, Edith, and Joyce at a pub in Staffordshire, which is half-way for both of us to travel. We had a nice Sunday lunch, but needless to say I was tired again when we got home at about 4.30pm. I had a quiet evening and another early night ready for the busy week ahead.

Friday 14th September

It is my birthday today. I always call it my "Happy Sad Day" as obviously Alan my twin would also have been celebrating if he had survived his cancer.

The day is quite memorable in an odd sort of way – I have an appointment at the Doctors to collect my prescription for the oestrogen blocking drug and then radiotherapy in the afternoon. Not a very normal birthday. Colleagues from work surprised me by sending me a bunch of flowers, as I haven't been in work since Wednesday morning. (I am only working three mornings during this treatment period). They are kind and thoughtful. Andy took me out for a quiet meal in the evening to celebrate.

Radiotherapy has been a mixture of journeys this week – if they keep me waiting then the journey can become three hours in total. If I am in quickly it is just over two hours in total.

Sunday 16th September

Yesterday was a very different day – no Queen Elizabeth

radiotherapy visit for one thing! In the morning we went to a leather shop to buy a new leather jacket for my birthday present. Andy chose to buy me two different jackets, as they are both lovely and it would have been really hard to have chosen between them. I was amazed when he suggested it and the reason he gave was, 'Because I love you and you are worth it.' He is wonderful and we really are much stronger and closer, as a result of the last few months.

In the evening we went to Andy and Karon's for an Abba pop group theme evening. Making the costumes and deciding what to wear took me ages during the week – as if I hadn't got enough to think about really. The evening was one long laugh from start to finish. It was one o'clock in the morning when I went to bed. Hence I am rather tired today. I am usually okay at the time but it does catch up with me and nearly always the next day.

Wednesday 19th September

The last two days have been tiring, as I have been at work from 8.30am until 1.00pm. I have then driven for 25 minutes to get home to meet Andy. He has taken me to radiotherapy. The waiting time has been between 40 minutes to 52 minutes, so yesterday (the worst day) we left home at 2.30pm and walked back in at 5.10pm. Needless to say once I have cooked tea, eaten it and cleared away, I am then off to bed really early. Then today I went in within seconds of arriving and the total time was two hours and 15 minutes, which is reasonably manageable.

Thursday 20th September

I went to see the Oncologist at 9.00am again. He is happy with my progress but did make the comment, 'Don't do too much.' I had mentioned how tired I was this morning after three mornings of work plus travelling to radiotherapy. He is right really – it is only three weeks since the last dose of chemotherapy so it will still be in my body. I have had surgery, returned to work and I am now tackling the daily grind of radiotherapy visits. I am philosophically taking one day at a time, but it must all take its' toll on my stamina. This spell is relentless, especially the travel, but today is session twelve so we are now over half-way through. Roll on 4th October.

Friday 21st September

I drove to the wig shop this morning. I wear my wig all the time and wash it by hand once a week to keep it in condition. I have noticed that the clips at the side, which grip my head, seem loose and the wig has lost some of the original sheen and appears a bit flat. I decided to telephone the wig shop for advice. The assistant said that as I had worn it full-time for six months it was actually getting worn out as that is their life expectancy. She advised me to buy another one. Andy and I discussed whether I should have the same again or choose a shorter style as a transition to emerging from under the wig. I have decided to have the same again, as I don't think I want another new look at the moment. People make such a fuss when they see you with a new look. I have been through enough already really without making my life anymore complicated. It cost me £130 but I feel it is such a saviour for my lifestyle and makes me feel so good about myself that it has to be worth spending to gain so many advantages.

Sunday 23rd September

It has been a quiet restful weekend to recharge my batteries ready for work and more radiotherapy. It is such a welcome break not to go to hospital at weekends. Andy has decided he will start to decorate the living room, which we haven't done for about ten years. He has been stripping wallpaper and moving electric sockets. He finds such projects very relaxing compared with his daily job. I think he also finds it a distraction from the worries my illness has placed upon us both.

Thursday 27th September

I went to see the Oncologist again for my weekly check. He took one look at my breasts and said 'Brilliant skin, doing very well indeed'. Apparently some patients get soreness, redness and cracked skin. My skin is totally normal at the moment and you wouldn't think I was on radiotherapy at this stage. He used a felt pen to mark a cross about two inches big along my scar and at right angles to it. This is ready for the last two localised boosts of radiotherapy next week (final two!). All other doses have been to treat the whole breast area.

I had another three-hour plus round trip today because of having to wait an hour to be seen. It is so very tiring and when I am driving it makes it worse. Andy is wonderful; he has taken me Monday to Wednesday every week and then I have taken myself on Thursdays and Fridays. He has walked Chloe all week, as I am tired when we get home between 5.00pm and 6.00pm. I am regularly in bed by 8.30pm or 9.00pm.

I am still wearing my wonderful wig. My hair is growing quicker now that I am getting out of the chemotherapy treatment cycle. It isn't very long though and definitely not long enough for me to feel comfortable being seen without my wig. It is interesting seeing the other radiotherapy patients in the hospital waiting area. You can definitely tell which ones have just finished chemotherapy, as their hair is like a crew cut and very short indeed. Many of them look gaunt and quite ill really – maybe they are – I don't know. I do know that I look as though I haven't had any chemo at all and still look very well, as my skin is clear and I am still managing to smile most of the time - well at least in public!

I am beginning to get a bit concerned about my weight. I

have remained the same weight throughout my treatment so far and not moved in any direction – up or down. I am now five pounds heavier than I was a month ago and some of my clothes are staring to feel a bit tight. I wonder if it is the oestrogen blocker tablets as one of the side effects can be weight gain. I didn't particularly want this to happen as I think I am heavy enough as it is, and I am now the heaviest I have ever been in my life. I'll talk to the Oncologist about it next week.

Saturday 29th September

A break from radiotherapy treatment today; only four more sessions to go now. I can't wait to get rid of the journey and obviously the treatment too. Next Thursday is the end of nearly nine months continuous treatment – no wonder it takes at least three to six months to get your stamina and energy back. We are off for a Thai meal tonight with friends Barry and Lillian. It should be really good.

I feel a bit fragile as I've been for a monthly chiropractor visit and he did several manipulations to my joints. I will have to be careful for a few days to give it time to settle down. Another frustration – it is one thing or another – it will be good to feel well one day.

Tuesday 2nd October

Only two more to go! I have finished all 20 treatments of

the whole breast area. They were not too late with the appointments today so it was two and a half hours total, which is a bit more reasonable – but still most of the afternoon and still tiring.

I am so weary this week. We had a late night Saturday and also the last few weeks are catching up with me. Tiredness is one of the side effects. Andy and I can't wait to finish the horrendous daily round trips.

Relief and exhaustion

Thursday 4th October

It seems a long time since my first visit to the doctors on January 24th and the start of nearly nine months continuous treatment. Today is a true milestone and celebration, as it is the end of the treatment – apart from my daily tablet for the next five years. It feels strange and surreal but we are both so relieved to get the daily travelling finished.

For the last two radiotherapy sessions they have used a special device - a sort of square frame to ensure that it is only focussed upon the scar area. They said it is to catch any rogue cancer cells. I have always believed that the cancer went after the surgery, therefore such comments seem both odd and alien to me. I hope I am right and they did go then.

We opened a bottle of champagne and had just one glass each to celebrate. We are both driving to work in the morning. I am so proud of myself and so is Andy. Karon rang me and sent me a text message, as she is really pleased for me. It has been a long haul up Mount Everest but I can still see the Christmas lights at the top. It will take me some months now to build up my stamina and energy, and probably be the New Year before I begin to feel anything like normal again.

My weight has increased by half a stone since the end of August and I don't feel good about it. The Oncologist seemed to think it was probably my tablets and not to worry about it. I suppose I shouldn't worry providing I am reasonably fit and well and the cancer is under control. It is going to take some controlling and but I think at the moment I am not going to start dieting as I just can't face the regime after the last nine months. Andy says he still loves me, which is important to me.

Sunday 7th October

One thing I can't get used to is the fact I have no medical appointments for another three weeks when I will see the Oncologist again. It seems strange after the relentless appointment regime over the last six weeks.

We had a super Cantonese meal with Andy and Karon, and Bob and Dot last night. We invited them to celebrate with us and they certainly spoilt me with lovely gifts including an "In the pink" t-shirt and some sexy underwear. I wonder if it will have any affect on Andy.

Dad, Edith and Joyce travelled down from Nantwich today. It is Dad's 79th birthday, so it was a double celebration weekend. We went out for lunch to save cooking. I was tired when they left at 6.30pm. Dad and Edith seem to enjoy each other's company and have just returned from a five-day break in Wales. He seems relaxed about me, including my future health prognosis. We've all just got to get on with life and only time will prove if the prognosis and outcome results in another 20 to 30 years with Andy. I do hope so. I don't think anyone who hasn't suffered cancer and experienced the tough treatment, and the way cancer is life threatening, could actually comprehend how I feel. The thought of death is absolutely horrendous when I allow it to bubble to the surface and find a chink in my armour.

Thursday 11th October

I am at home today as part of my two days off work. It seems strange being at home and still part-time now that I have finished treatment. I feel a bit of a fraud really but I am not well enough to work full-time at the moment and intend building up to be full-time in the spring.

I feel absolutely exhausted and washed out, which is compounded by a huge relief that nearly nine months of relentless treatment is suddenly over. I am so low on power and stamina. It is going to take months to build it up, feel fit, and full of energy.

My right breast is pink in colour and has soreness underneath, which is where my bra rubs if I wear one for work. I haven't been wearing a bra whilst at home, as advised by the radiotherapy team. I think it has helped. Even though I finished treatment last Thursday the tiredness and soreness can continue for more than two weeks. I also still can't use soap and antiperspirant in the area for the next fortnight. The regime continues on...

Sunday 14th October

It has been a busy weekend. We enjoyed a carvery meal at a pub on Friday evening before going to an amateur dramatic production with Andy and Karon. They are proud of me and still praise me for how well I have tackled and coped with the treatment.

On Saturday evening Liz and Richard visited us for a meal. It was a pleasant evening and a reasonably easy meal to prepare and cook. It was after midnight when we went to bed. Andy was tired but our alarm clock went off at 5.30am for him to be collected by taxi at 6.45am to be driven to Heathrow airport. It was an early start for a long trip to India on business again. He will be back on Thursday night. I have had a quiet Sunday with Chloe and have been able to rest a lot ready for my five hours of work again tomorrow.

Thursday 18th October

I have been busy with part-time work and lots of dog walking whilst Andy has been away. I have managed well but I am getting tired and still feel low on stamina. I ended up at the doctors - it must be withdrawal systems! I had an ear blocked with wax and had to have the wax removed by a syringe. One day I might feel really fit and well again.

Andy is due back tonight and I am looking forward to seeing him as I miss him tremendously. Chloe does too. Mo continues to walk Chloe with me most days in the week. We have become good friends and she is a great positive mentor for me.

Sunday 21st October

We have had a busy but pleasant weekend enjoying each other's company now Andy is home from India. He was tired after all of the travelling and rested at home on Friday as time-in-lieu, which is company policy.

We enjoyed a wine tasting evening with some of the neighbours. Again they are all concerned and kind hearted, asking me how I am and praising me for how I seem to have been over the months. Obviously they don't always appreciate nor comprehend the real side effects that you have to constantly deal with. Many of them seem surprised at how well I am looking – again that expectation that cancer patients usually don't look well during treatment.

Tuesday 23rd October

I have worked two days at the start of the school half-term holiday. I will then be on leave for three days. We are travelling to Wales on Thursday morning for two nights in our favourite hotel. Chloe will go with us. It will stop us doing jobs at home, e.g. decorating the living room, and give us some quality time together. I have an appointment with the Oncologist on Thursday morning when I think he will discharge me and hand me back to progress visits with the Consultant for Breast Surgery.

Saturday 27th October

We have returned from Wales today after a lovely restful break. We feel as though we are both coming up for air after eight and half months of treatment. It is going to take a long time to feel fully fit and on track again. Walking was limited, but better than walking and touring on holiday in August. I was disappointed not to be able to visit Nantwich to put flowers on Mum's grave for her birthday yesterday. It is also my sister-in-law Gill's birthday today, so I sent her some flowers. She is Alan's widow and has been through a lot herself.

It was good news on Thursday when I kept my nine

o'clock appointment with the Oncologist before we travelled to Wales. He was delighted with my recovery from the radiotherapy and told me that I could start to use soap and antiperspirant again. Thank goodness. He discharged me from his care as expected. Whilst I was waiting to see him in the small cubicles outside his consulting room, I was chatting to a man and his wife. She had been diagnosed with breast cancer and was about to start chemotherapy after her surgery. She was keen to ask me how well I had been and felt reassured by some of my comments. They were very worried about the hair loss side-effect and were amazed when I informed them that my hair was a wig. They said it was so natural and they really had no idea. She stated how much more positive she felt having seen my healthy state and fabulous wig. I certainly owe a lot to this wig and my determination to beat this *'bugger'*.

Wednesday 31st October

I have just returned from my monthly visit to the chiropractor to keep on top of my joint problems. My aches and pains aren't too bad considering what I have been through all year and the fact I stopped attending the gym at the rehab clinic once I was diagnosed.

Andy is working hard in his spare time to try and complete the decorating of the living room, which has been going on for quite a while. We will get the house on track someday! It has been a tough few years with Mum's illness and now my illness. We are now at least on the right side of it all.

Sunday 4th November

Roger and Kate were due to join us for a meal last night but had to cancel. It meant we had a quiet weekend with nothing on socially. I decided to go shopping for some bits and to start Christmas shopping. I knew my stamina would be limited but I was washed out after just an hour. It took me a couple of hours to rest and recover. This is so frustrating, as I am beginning to feel less tired, much more like myself, and yet the stamina level is still an inhibitor.

Saturday 10th November

I have had a busy, mentally demanding few days this week and it has taken its' toll today. I look like I have worked a 50 to 60-hour week, like I used to do before I was ill. I had worked two and a half days consecutively with training and presentations to deliver, including lots of high concentration meetings. It has proved how I need to build up my stamina and mental concentration capacity, but most of all that I am not ready to work 8.30am to 5.00pm every day. I obviously need to take my time building up and also continue to get early nights.

Andy had to clear the furniture in the living room and

lift the carpet on Thursday evening. The new carpet was fitted yesterday and the wallpapering is well on the way. We are still in a mess; which could get me down if I let it!

Friday 16th November

Andy has now finished the wall papering in the evenings this week and the curtains are being fitted tomorrow. At last we are getting the room back.

I ended up working for three full days and on the other two days of this week until 10.00am or 10.30am. I had to swap things around to attend a curriculum design workshop on Thursday. It is connected with an aspect of my job that I am leading on as did the meeting on Tuesday morning. I've had to make sure I had lots of rest in between and not be too late to bed. I am usually in bed now between 9.00pm and 9.45pm, which is later than my usual 8.00pm when I was on a chemotherapy treatment.

Sunday 18th November

We had dinner at Bob and Dot's last night. Andy and Karon were there too so it was great to see everyone. They were saying how much better I am looking – although I have never looked terrible – especially whilst wearing my wonderful wig!

Thursday 22nd November

I have been out for lunch today at a local pub. I met Barbara who is one of my colleagues, who retired last summer, and now works two days a week on specific projects. She is kind and thoughtful, and has emailed me regularly from the start. She lost her first husband from cancer so understands some of the impact and side effects. It was a lovely lunch and chat, which is good for me.

The living room is finally finished and we are both delighted with it. It is very different and much more modern too.

I am getting fed up with my hair taking so long to grow – it is probably about an inch or three centimetres long but very uneven. I feel a bit boxed in by my wig. It is so good and does suit me, which means I am now reluctant to let go of it until I feel comfortable. I suppose there is no right or wrong way of dealing with it. I have made an appointment with Lisa my hairdresser for Sunday 23rd December – will I be ready to emerge by then? I'm not sure.

Sunday 25th November

We went to Nantwich last night to see Dad and Joyce. Edith was away on holiday for a week so we didn't see her this time. We went to the local pub for a superb good value meal and a chat. Dad and Joyce seem well and Dad is very positive about my progress. He also thinks I am looking better and less tired. He obviously still enjoys Edith's company and they spend a lot of time together, which is good for both of them.

I have finished planning a 'Pink Party,' which I am hosting at home next Saturday. It has given me something to focus upon and is a means of saying thank you to our friends who have been extremely supportive throughout this year. I sent them invitations a few weeks ago and there will be 18 of us in total. Unfortunately Wendy and Clive, Liz and Richard, and Barry and Lillian can't make it due to other arrangements. I intend holding a raffle in aid of Breakthrough Breast Cancer – none of us know when we will need the latest and best treatment – it could be next week as I discovered in February.

Friday 30th November

I am not at work today as I have worked four days already this week. I went shopping for the party food on my way home last night. It was easier than turning out again today. I intend tidying the house and preparing some of the food today. Dave and Jayne are also arriving on Saturday afternoon to stay overnight with us. Dave was our best man 30 years ago and they live in Cheshire.

Monday 3rd December

I am absolutely exhausted from the party and the preparation I had to do, even though I tried to make things easy for myself. Andy helped tremendously; and Dave and Jayne were also marvellous. Our 18 wonderful friends arrived and we had a great evening together celebrating our friendship. They are amazingly generous as several brought gifts for the raffle and we raised £120 from the draw. It was one laugh after another and I think everyone thoroughly enjoyed it. I certainly did and was very touched by their generosity – I had difficulty telling them the amount as I was nearly in tears. Many of them helped to clear away and wash up which meant I had very little to do when they went home. Karon, Bella and Jayne were fantastic and so busy in the kitchen, as well as keeping their eye on me. They are great friends and anyone going through this ordeal and journey through the relentless treatment needs to remember the value of friendship.

Christmas lights at the top of Mount Everest

Saturday 8th December

I undertook a one-day review of a subject department in a secondary school this week. It is always a very busy, mentally demanding day, even when working alongside another colleague. I coped much better than I thought I would, which was a positive outcome. I was tired but not as bad as I expected after the solid concentration from 8.30am until 5.00pm with lots of judgements to make throughout.

We have had a quiet weekend after such a busy one last weekend. I did some Christmas shopping for 50 minutes at a Retail Park on my way home. I made good progress and it wasn't too busy as it was rush hour time and people were going home instead of shopping. I only had to go into two stores and parked outside, so it wasn't as demanding as wandering around can be for me at this stage in my recovery. It is still frustrating to be less energetic than I used to be before my cancer.

Wednesday 12th December

I have been getting more and more worried and stressed since last Friday evening. I think my armpit area, where my lymph nodes were removed, feels different and slightly swollen, as though it is lumpier too. My breast is also a bit tender on the top and it feels as if the nerve tingles when I touch it. I have got very concerned that it is the cancer returned – but I can't believe that is possible only eight weeks after finishing months of treatment. It is a horrible feeling and no one else would understand unless they have had cancer themselves. I hope I am imagining it and just being silly now I am 'out on my own' without regular checks from the Oncologist. The problem is that I thought I was silly and neurotic last time and we all know what happened then!

I telephoned the Consultant Breast Care Nurse who reassured me it was unlikely to be a major problem so soon after all the treatment. It could be lymphoedema starting, or an after effect of the radiotherapy. She has agreed to see me on Friday afternoon so I feel a bit more relaxed now. I just want her to tell me I am silly and to go home.

Friday 14th December

I am so very relieved, as she has told me that the lumpiness is a side effect of the radiotherapy and could be around for up to a year. I am so pleased and totally chilled tonight. I just can't explain how scary it was to think it could be secondary cancer. I feel a bit silly about the panic, but I know I have done the right thing getting it checked. I need to keep an eye on things, know my body, but also have the confidence to get on with my life too – a fine balancing act. Andy is extremely relieved and as supportive and positive as ever. They did an ultrasound scan and it was all clear of cancer, which is reassuring. I have my three-month check-up with the Consultant on the morning of New Year's Eve. I hope and believe it will all be OK and we can say Goodbye to 2007 in style.

Thursday 20th December

I am very tired today as I have been out for two evenings as well as working during the day. On Tuesday the Advisers team went out for a Christmas meal. It was a very pleasant end to a tough term. On Wednesday I attended the Awards Ceremony at one of the secondary schools. It has been good to be getting back into schools during this half term and work directly with teachers, which is the aspect of the job that I enjoy the most.

We all finish for Christmas tomorrow and I am definitely on my last legs with stamina and mental tiredness. It has been an extremely difficult school term with the radiotherapy treatment, surgery to remove the implant device, and finishing chemotherapy; all just at the time when the pupils returned to schools. Some rest time will be really appreciated.

Sunday 23rd December

Today has been stressful and emotional for me. I was very nervous driving to the hair salon, as I felt as if I was going for an interview for a new job. Fortunately Lisa took me into the shampoo area where I could sit at the mirror and around the corner from the main salon section. There was one lady waiting to have her hair washed and the teenager who washes customers' hair when I took a deep breath and removed my wig. I was petrified really at the thought of removing my wig in a public place, because only Andy and the lady in the wig suppliers have ever seen me without it. I had taken a carrier bag with me and very quickly placed my wig in it so from then onwards I looked like any other customer in the salon.

Lisa was surprised how long my hair was (about one-and-half inches or seven centimetres) and we decided to highlight it to add thickness, colour and life. I am not sure if it was too early for adding colour or not but we decided to anyway. She cut it extremely well into a short tussled style that you use your fingers to ruffle. When I got home – after the really strange experience of walking to my car and driving home without the wig – Andy was very surprised how good the haircut looked. He instantly said, 'Go for it. The wig should be history.' I think I agree.

Mo, my friend and neighbour, came round to see how I had got on. It was sweet of her, as she knew what a major step it was for me to decide to emerge from under the wig. She also agreed with Andy and told me to forget the wig. I took another deep breath and thought – go for it girl!

I have worn my wig for nine months and it has been my saviour for normality and a quality of life. I have never walked out of the house without it and have even worn a scarf when I have gone downstairs in my dressing gown or to fetch something in my pyjamas. I decided before I went to the hairdressers that my pink and black designer glasses would be quite heavy with a very short hairstyle. I had talked to Andy about it and decided that the finer deep purple-framed glasses maybe better to wear for the next few months until my hair grows and thickens out more. I took them with me in my handbag and changed glasses before I walked out of the salon. I might as well have lots of change at once.

It feels very cold around the back of my head – especially when I walked Chloe this afternoon in the country lanes with the December wind blowing. It has been a huge day, but a necessary step in moving on. I have now got to face family, friends, and work colleagues with another new look and all their comments. The impact of having cancer and the treatment is never ending and people don't